BANISH *Your* BELLY
Butt & Thighs
in 30 Days!

By the Editors of *PREVENTION.* Magazine

RODALE

© 2001 by Rodale Inc.

Printed in the United States of America

The straight leg lift and inner thigh lift on page 145 and the opposite arm and leg lift on page 146 were reprinted with permission from Miriam Nelson, Ph.D. She is the associate chief of the physiology laboratory at Tufts University in Boston and author of the international bestsellers *Strong Women Stay Young* (Bantam, 2000) and *Strong Women Stay Slim* (Bantam, 1998). Her latest book is *Strong Women, Strong Bones* (Putnam, 2000).

ISBN 1–57954–525–4   paperback

2 4 6 8 10 9 7 5 3 1   paperback

Visit us on the Web at www.rodalestore.com, or call us toll-free at (800) 848-4735.

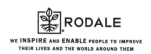

WE INSPIRE AND ENABLE PEOPLE TO IMPROVE
THEIR LIVES AND THE WORLD AROUND THEM

Prevention *Banish Your Belly, Butt, and Thighs in 30 Days!* Staff

EDITOR
Bridget Doherty

WRITERS
Kristine Napier, R.D.; Kim Galeaz, R.D.;
Roberta Duyff, R.D.; Elizabeth Ward, R.D.;
Betsy Bates; Judith Lin Eftekhar; Susan Huxley;
Holly McCord, R.D.

INTERIOR AND COVER DESIGNER
Carol Angstadt

PHOTO EDITOR
Robin Hepler

SENIOR COPY EDITOR
Karen Neely

EDITORIAL PRODUCTION MANAGER
Marilyn Hauptly

LAYOUT DESIGNER
Jennifer H. Giandomenico

MANUFACTURING COORDINATORS
Brenda Miller, Jodi Schaffer, Patrick T. Smith

Rodale Women's Health Group

VICE PRESIDENT, EDITORIAL DIRECTOR
Elizabeth Crow

PREVENTION **EDITOR-IN-CHIEF**
Catherine Cassidy

EDITOR-IN-CHIEF, WOMEN'S HEALTH BOOKS
Tammerly Booth

PREVENTION **SPECIAL INTEREST PUBLICATIONS
EXECUTIVE EDITOR**
Cindi Caciolo

SENIOR EDITOR, WOMEN'S HEALTH BOOKS
Sharon Faelten

PREVENTION **BUSINESS MANAGER**
Frank Dragotta

MANAGING EDITOR
Madeleine Adams

ART DIRECTOR
Darlene Schneck

RESEARCH DIRECTOR
Ann Gossy Yermish

MANAGER OF CONTENT ASSEMBLY
Robert V. Anderson Jr.

DIGITAL PROCESSING GROUP MANAGERS
Leslie M. Keefe, Thomas P. Aczel

PRODUCT DIRECTOR
Dan Shields

MANUFACTURING MANAGER
Eileen Bauder

OFFICE STAFF
Julie Kehs Minnix, Catherine E. Strouse

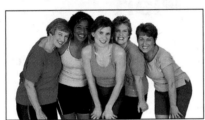

CONTENTS

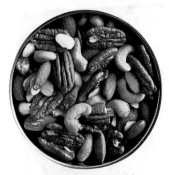

FAT BLASTER:
Learn the truth
about nuts
PAGE 5

PART 1
The Body-Shaping Menu Plan

PART 2
The 30-Day Shape-Up Plan

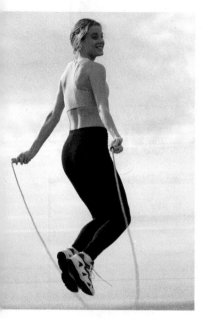

FAT BLASTER:
The best ways to
jump rope
PAGE 100

iv

PART 3
Shape-Up Success—Guaranteed

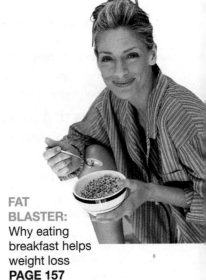

FAT BLASTER:
Why eating breakfast helps weight loss
PAGE 157

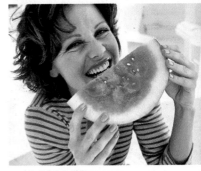

FAT BLASTER:
Banish bad eating habits—for good
PAGE 187

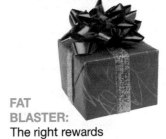

FAT BLASTER:
The right rewards spell S-U-C-C-E-S-S
PAGE 196

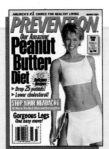

Editorial Advisors

Rosemary Agostini, M.D., primary-care sports medicine physician at the Virginia Mason Sports Medicine Center and clinical associate professor of orthopedics at the University of Washington, both in Seattle

Barbara D. Bartlik, M.D., clinical assistant professor in the department of psychiatry at Weill Medical College of Cornell University and assistant attending psychiatrist at the New York–Presbyterian Hospital, both in New York City

Mary Ruth Buchness, M.D., chief of dermatology at St. Vincent's Hospital and Medical Center in New York City and associate professor of dermatology and medicine at the New York Medical College in Valhalla

Leah J. Dickstein, M.D., professor and associate chairperson for academic affairs in the department of psychiatry and behavioral sciences and associate dean for faculty and student advocacy at the University of Louisville School of Medicine in Kentucky and past president of the American Medical Women's Association (AMWA)

Jean L. Fourcroy, M.D., Ph.D., past president of the American Medical Women's Association (AMWA) and of the National Council on Women's Health

JoAnn E. Manson, M.D., Dr.P.H., professor of medicine at Harvard Medical School and chief of preventive medicine at Brigham and Women's Hospital in Boston

Terry L. Murphy, Psy.D., assistant clinical professor in the department of community health and aging at Temple University and a licensed clinical psychologist in Philadelphia

Susan C. Olson, Ph.D., clinical psychologist, life transition/psychospiritual therapist, and weight-management consultant in Seattle

Mary Lake Polan, M.D., Ph.D., professor and chairperson of the department of gynecology and obstetrics at Stanford University School of Medicine

Lila Amdurska Wallis, M.D., M.A.C.P., clinical professor of medicine at Weill Medical College of Cornell University in New York City, past president of the American Medical Women's Association (AMWA), founding president of the National Council on Women's Health, director of continuing medical education programs for physicians, and master and laureate of the American College of Physicians

Carla Wolper, R.D., nutritionist and clinical coordinator at the Obesity Research Center at St. Luke's–Roosevelt Hospital Center and nutritionist at the Center for Women's Health at Columbia-Presbyterian/Eastside, both in New York City

SHOP _PREVENTION_!

PRODUCT

ITEM	NUMBER	PRICE	QTY.	TOTAL
▶ **Prevention's Fat to Firm in 20 Minutes!** A total-body, strength training workout video	052400	$15.95		
Master the Slender Life A 12-part weight loss planner	051131	$7.00		
Fit & Firm Workout A step-by-step guide to strength training	051521	$5.00		
▶ **Prevention's Personal Health Advisor** A 64-page woman's self-assessment guide for optimum health	PHA01	$4.95		
"Take a Walk Today" Audiotape (Availability limited) Moderate walking pace with encouragement from Walking Editor Maggie Spilner	AV2	$10.95		
▶ **Banish Your Belly, Butt & Thighs** Get fit, firm, and fabulous—forever! The real woman's guide to body shaping & weight loss	BYBBT1	$29.95		
Easy Measure Calipers **and Instructional Pamphlet** The efficient and practical way to measure your body fat percentage utilizing skinfold measurement	CAL01	$12.00		
▶ **Prevention's Fat to Fit Video** Our new energizing aerobic workout for all levels	VIDO2	$16.95		

Subtotal	$	
Handling Charge	$ 3.00	
(CA, CO, GA, IL, MI, NY, PA please include applicable sales tax)	$	
TOTAL (US Dollars)	$	

NEW VIDEO!

To Order, Call (800) 325-3186

ORDERED BY (please print)

Name

Address

City/State

Zip/Postal Code

Payment Method: Check or Money Order☐   Visa ☐   Mastercard ☐   Amex ☐   Discover ☐

Credit Card # ☐☐☐☐☐☐☐☐☐☐☐☐☐☐☐☐   SZ0101

Expiration Date ☐☐ ☐☐   **Cardholder's Signature**

Please make your check or money order payable to **Prevention Magazine.** Send this form (or a copy) and your payment to Shop Prevention, P.O. Box 1120, Ronks, PA 17573. Allow 6 to 8 weeks for delivery. Thank you!

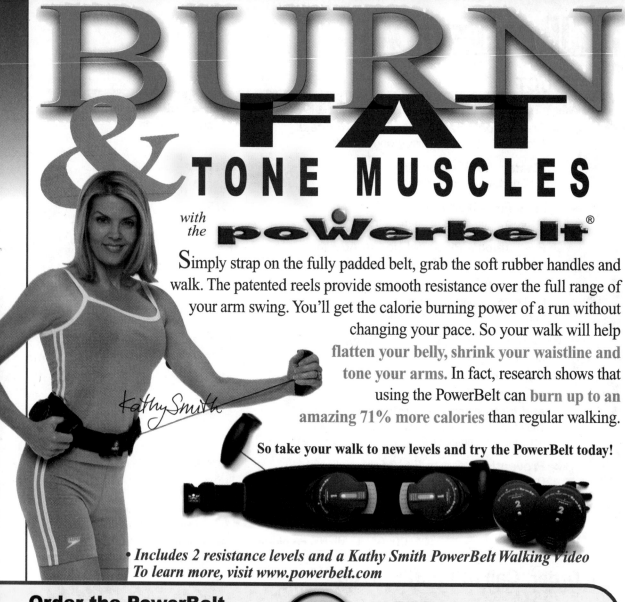

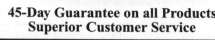

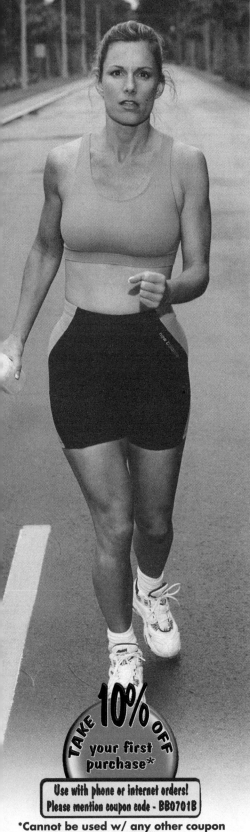
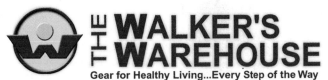

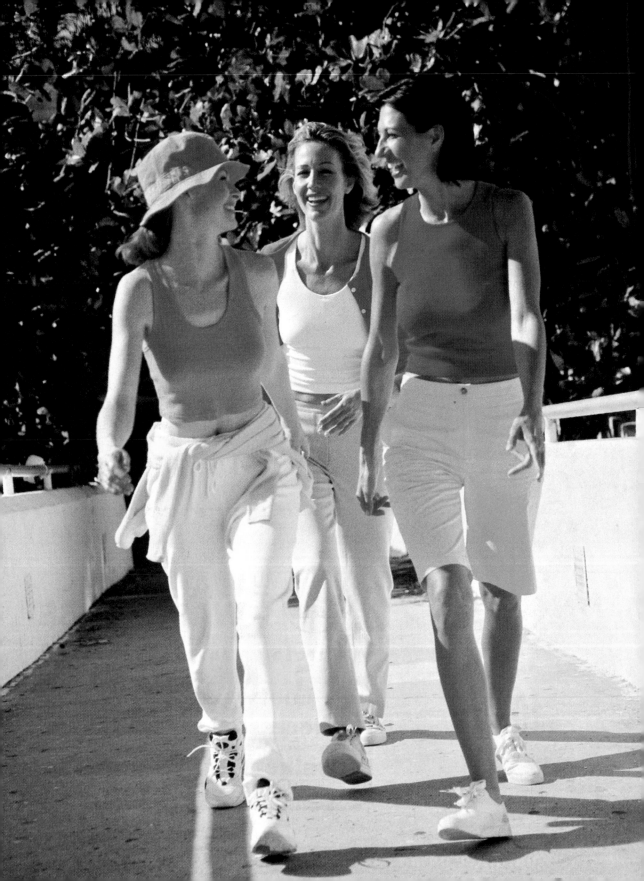

Introduction

Finally . . . A Plan You Can Live With!

It's time to stop letting a bulging belly, saggy behind, or jiggly thighs ruin your day! Think about how much power you're giving one measly body part when you stand in front of the mirror, scold yourself for not being perfect, and then pull out the dark-colored baggy clothes to hide behind.

You need to take back that power and put it to better use—shaping up those trouble spots! With this program, it's possible. And I'll be right there with you, working off my post-pregnancy pounds and getting back my prebaby belly.

What makes this program so successful is that you can customize it to meet your needs. If the most exercise you're used to getting is lapping the grocery store aisle, you can start with the beginner workouts. That way you'll avoid one of the most common beginner mistakes—doing too much too soon—which can sideline you with injuries or leave you hating exercise. And we'll show you 26 fun ways to burn off calories and tone your particular trouble spot.

No weight-loss program would be complete without a healthy diet. But this program does more than just give you a "one-size-fits-all" meal plan. The 150 Fat-Blasting Foods can help you develop a shopping list of low-fat, flavorful foods that will help you to shed pounds. But if you prefer something a little more regimented, we have the 7-Day Quick-Start Menu. Best of all, you can enjoy your favorites—even if it is chocolate—and still lose weight.

Most important, you'll feel good while you slim down. In addition to inspirational stories from average women who've succeeded, you'll learn how to stop the negative self-talk that can sabotage your efforts; how to dress to look two sizes smaller, even before you drop a pound; and how to stay motivated. After years of coaching women, I've found that it's easier to get back into shape when you feel good about yourself.

Turn the page and watch your trouble spots disappear.

Michele Stanten

Michele Stanten
Fitness Editor
Prevention Magazine

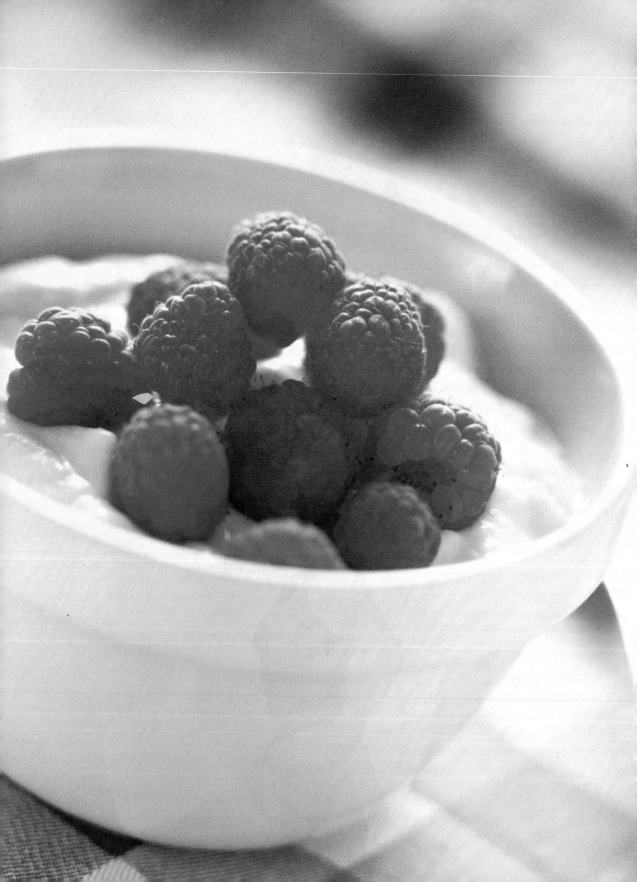

Part 1

The Body-Shaping Menu Plan

Chapter 1

The Banish Your Belly, Butt, and Thighs Diet

Lose all the weight you want— *and* protect your health!

Tired of hearing about the high-protein diet, the grapefruit diet, the eat-while-standing-on-your-head diet? All these diets may promise the world, but you know you could never eat this way your whole life. You want the perfect plan that you can live with forever. Well, look no further. The Banish Your Belly, Butt, and Thighs Diet is here! It's a simple-to-use meal plan that features regular foods. We've designed it to deliver 1,500 to 1,600 calories a day, a gradual-weight-loss diet for most women.

Another bonus: Studies show that the foods in this diet should lower your risk of heart attack, osteoporosis, high blood pressure, cancer, stroke, diabetes, cataracts, diverticulosis, obesity, depression, and even PMS.

To make it even easier, we've devised the Banish Your Belly, Butt, and Thighs 30-Day Planner on page 148, which includes an easy-to-use checklist to help you keep track. Start with these nine steps today!

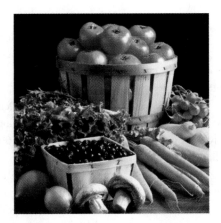

and cancers. If you've been eating a high-carbohydrate diet with lots of refined grains, typically breads, rolls, bagels, pretzels, and crackers made from white flour, it may be a challenge at first to find whole grain substitutes.

But the payoff is worth it. To your body, refined white flour is the same as sugar, making a diet high in white-flour foods the same as a high-sugar diet. Start reading the ingredient lists of all of your grain products. Choose the ones made with a whole grain; you should see the actual word "whole."

Step 1

Eat nine servings of vegetables and fruits every day.

Veggies and fruits are the foundation of the Banish Your Belly, Butt, and Thighs Diet—as opposed to grains, the foundation of the traditional Food Guide Pyramid. Eat nine ½-cup servings of a variety of fruits and veggies every day. Does that sound like overkill? In reality, it could mean extra life. Study after study links diets highest in fruits and vegetables with fewer cancers and less heart disease, diabetes, and even osteoporosis. The landmark DASH (Dietary Approaches to Stop Hypertension) diet study found that nine servings a day lowered blood pressure as much as some prescription drugs.

More experts agree that five vegetables and four fruits are the optimum. In our diet, you'll need to make every meal and snack a fruit or veggie opportunity.

Step 2

Eat three to six whole grain foods every day.

Diets high in whole grains are linked to less heart disease and diabetes and fewer strokes

---

What's a Serving?

Vegetables and Fruits
½ cup chopped fruit
½ cup cooked or raw veggies
1 cup raw green leafy veggies
¾ cup vegetable or fruit juice
1 medium piece of fruit

Whole Grains
1 slice whole wheat bread
½ cup brown rice or bulgur
½ cup whole wheat pasta

High-Calcium Foods
1 cup fat-free or 1% milk
1 cup fat-free or low-fat yogurt
1 cup calcium-fortified orange juice
1 ounce reduced-fat cheese

Beans
½ cup cooked dried beans/lentils

Nuts
2 tablespoons, chopped

Fish
3 ounces, cooked

Whole grains also mean extra fiber, the closest thing to a weight-loss magic bullet. Not only does it fill you up quickly with fewer calories, but it also eliminates some of the calories you eat! Fiber whisks calories through your system so quickly that some never have a chance to end up on your hips. To maximize fiber's slimming powers, aim for 25 to 35 grams a day. By eating 30 grams a day, your body will absorb almost 120 fewer calories daily.

Step 3

Eat two or three calcium-rich foods every day.

Calcium may lower your body fat. A group of women who ate at least 1,000 milligrams of calcium a day, along with a diet of no more than 1,900 calories daily, lost more weight—as much as 7 pounds more—than women who ate less calcium. It could be that calcium suppresses certain hormones, resulting in decreased fat production and increased fat breakdown. Not only does calcium support strong bones and help prevent osteoporosis, studies suggest that it helps prevent colon cancer, high blood pressure, and PMS as well.

If you're 50 or older or have low bone density, you should get 1,500 milligrams of calcium daily. If you're younger than 50, aim for 1,000 milligrams.

Obvious high-calcium choices include 1% and fat-free milk, low-fat and fat-free yogurt, and reduced-fat and fat-free cheese. Other good choices are orange and grapefruit juices and soy milk that have been fortified with calcium.

Step 4

Eat beans at least five times a week.

Beans are the highest-fiber foods you can find. Diets high in fiber are linked to less cancer, heart disease, and diabetes, and fewer strokes and even ulcers. And we've already told you what fiber can do for your weight-loss efforts.

Beans are the **highest-fiber** foods you can find.

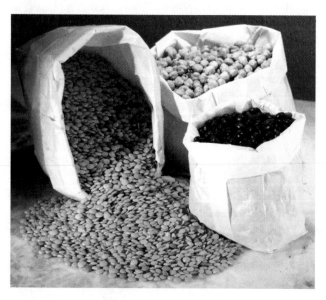

Beans are especially high in soluble fiber, which also lowers cholesterol levels, and folate, which lowers levels of yet another risk factor for heart disease: homocysteine.

Step 5

Nosh on nuts five times a week.

Studies show that people who eat nuts regularly have less heart disease and fewer other illnesses than people who avoid them. The key to eating nuts is to not eat too many; they're high in calories. To avoid temptation, keep a jar of chopped nuts in your fridge. Sprinkle 2 tablespoons a day on cereal, yogurt, veggies, salads, or wherever the crunch and rich flavor appeal to you.

FAT BLASTER

Be sure to store nuts in the refrigerator to keep them from oxidizing and turning rancid.

Step 6

Feast on fish twice a week.

Fish is an excellent source of protein because it's high in omega-3 fatty acids, which are good for your heart, while low in cholesterol and saturated fat. The protein in fish is a great hunger-stopper—and it helps build healthy muscles that burn tons of calories. To get the most omega-3s, choose salmon, white albacore tuna canned in water, rainbow trout, anchovies, herring, sardines, and mackerel.

FAT BLASTER

You can get a plant version of omega-3 fats in canola or flaxseed oil.

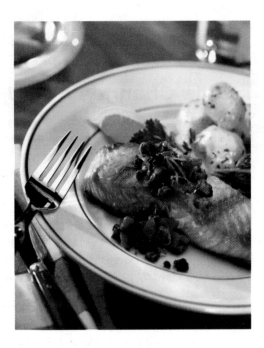

Step 7

Keep your fat budget.

To stay within a healthy fat budget—25 percent of calories from fat—you must first find the maximum fat allowance for your calorie level.

MAXIMUM FAT ALLOWANCE

Calories	Grams of Fat
1,250	35
1,500	42
1,750	49
2,000	56
2,250	63

Once you know your fat budget, see whether you're staying within the bounds by adding up the grams of fat for all the food that you eat in a day. Almost all food labels will tell you the grams of total fat in a serving. Try to get most of your fat from olive and canola oils

Real Women SHOW YOU HOW

Little Changes Add Up to 147 Pounds

A routine visit to the doctor 12 years ago changed Tammy Munson's life. She was diagnosed with alarmingly high blood pressure at the age of 21. Tammy weighed in at 253 pounds and, admittedly, knew little about nutrition. After her diagnosis, Tammy made two simple switches—from 2% milk to fat-free and from regular sodas to diet ones—and lost 30 pounds! After realizing how much her beverage choices affected her weight, Tammy began making better food choices, too. Within about a year, she had lost 147 pounds, and she has stayed at 106 pounds ever since.

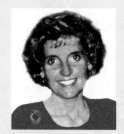

(or salad dressings made from them), trans-free margarine, nuts, and fish. And spread your fat throughout the day: A little fat with each meal helps you absorb fat-soluble nutrients from vegetables and fruits.

FAT BLASTER

To avoid trans fats, which raise cholesterol levels, avoid those products with the words "partially hydrogenated" in the ingredients list.

Step 8

Take some sensible nutrition insurance.

Besides your fabulous diet, take a multivitamin/mineral supplement, plus 100 to 400 IU of vitamin E and 100 to 500 milligrams of vitamin C daily. Also take 500 milligrams of calcium if you're under 50; take 1,000 milligrams of calcium (divided into two separate doses of 500 milligrams each) if you're 50 or older.

Step 9

Drink eight glasses of water every day, plus a cup or more of tea.

Every cell in your body needs water to function. And big water drinkers appear to get fewer colon and bladder cancers. Drinking lots of water helps you feel full, too. In addition, every cup of tea provides a strong infusion of antioxidants that help keep blood from clotting too easily (which may thwart heart attacks) and that may help lower your risk of cancer and rheumatoid arthritis.

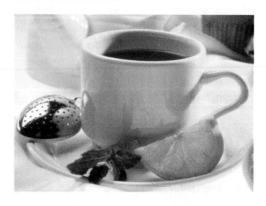

Chapter 2

150 Fat-Blasting Foods

The best foods that help you melt female fat and reshape your figure.

Burgers, desserts, cheese, tacos—believe it or not, these are fat-blasting foods! Under the Banish Your Belly, Butt, and Thighs program, the foods you love are the foods you can eat—and still lose weight. There's no living on carrot sticks and diet soda here. On the contrary, just about any food is game. You may be shocked to learn that foods you've been shunning aren't forbidden at all. "It's easier to stick to a healthful eating plan when you include some favorites," says Elizabeth Ward, R.D., a nutrition consultant in Stoneham, Massachusetts.

We've picked the best foods in each category so you don't have to do any work. Look up your favorite type of food, and you'll see the kinds you can eat, knowing that they'll help you drop pounds. To make things even easier, we added shopping tips that will help you know exactly what to buy so you can enjoy these foods and still cut out calories and fat.

BEST BAGELS, BREADS, ROLLS, AND MUFFINS

Bread Item	Portion	Calories	Grams of Fat
Whole grain bread	1 slice (1 oz)	70	1.1
Whole wheat pita	1 small pita (1 oz)	74	0.7
Tomato and basil tortilla	1 tortilla (1½ oz)	110	1.0
Low-fat blueberry muffin	1 muffin (2 oz)	162	6.2
Pumpernickel bagel	1 bagel (4 oz)	250	1.0

Shopping Smarts

For the bread you eat to qualify as the staff of life, you have to make the right choices when shopping. Here's what to look for.

Bread. Look for words like "100% whole wheat." ("Wheat bread" doesn't guarantee whole grain.) And check that some type of whole grain flour is listed as the first ingredient.

Bagels. Rather than grabbing a whole bag of one type, pick up one rye, one pumpernickel, one whole grain, one oat bran, and so forth. Even more important, pay attention to bagel size. Many bakery versions are the equivalent of five slices of bread and, at about 5 ounces, weigh in at around 390 calories.

Muffins. Beware. Some bakery muffins tip the scales at 15 grams of fat and 370 calories. Many fat-free ones are no calorie bargain either—the larger ones can weigh in with 350 to as many as 600 calories but very few nutrients.

Dinner rolls and biscuits. Some of the worst offenders are the ready-to-bake rolls and biscuits in the dairy case. Check the labels for fat and calories.

English muffins, French bread, and pita bread. These items tend to be very low in fat with a reasonable number of calories. Try to find whole wheat versions—even pitas now come in a variety of whole grain and vegetable mixes.

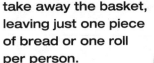

FAT BLASTER

In some restaurants, bread baskets rival the dessert cart. Ask the server to remove the butter. You might even want him to take away the basket, leaving just one piece of bread or one roll per person.

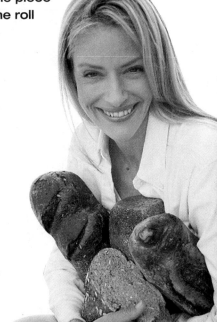

BEST BEVERAGES

Beverage	Serving Size	Calories	Grams of Fat
Still or sparkling water	8 oz	0	0.0
Unsweetened, flavored water	8 oz	0	0.0
Unsweetened, flavored iced tea	8 oz	5	0.0
Vegetable juice	8 oz	46	0.2
Calcium-fortified orange juice	8 oz	120	0.7
Grape juice	8 oz	127	0.2

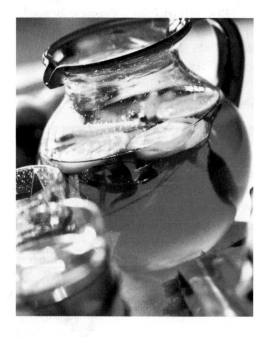

Shopping Smarts

For tips on buying milk and soy milk, see the "Shopping Smarts" section for milk and dairy on page 26. Otherwise, follow these purchasing tips.

Water. Given that water has zero fat and calories and can keep you from overeating, bottled water should appear on every grocery list. Buy enough for a week.

Still water is fine. If a little fizz helps you chug down more wet stuff, buy calorie-free flavored seltzer or club sodas. Just avoid the ones that are heavy in sugar and calories. They hide nearly as many calories as regular soda.

Coffee and coffee drinks. True, coffee contributes only 5 calories—if you drink it black. The real damage, however, comes from specialty coffees—the lattes, mochas, cappuccinos, and other tall treats sold in coffee bars and shops (and even some gas stations).

Iced tea. If you're going to drink iced tea, drink plain old-fashioned iced tea—made from tea bags and flavored with lemon. It has just 2 calories, plus you get plenty of water in the bargain.

Juices. With few exceptions, juice is mainly sugar. Two exceptions are calcium-fortified orange juice and vegetable juice.

FAT BLASTER

Sugar-free powdered beverages are blossoming in many flavors—from pedestrian lemonade to peach, raspberry, and strawberry flavor explosions. Mix up a pitcher year-round and keep it in the fridge to satisfy a sweet tooth.

BEST BURGERS AND HOT DOGS

Burger or Hot Dog	Portion	Calories	Grams of Fat
Fat-free hot dog	1 hot dog	40	0.0
Turkey hot dog	1 hot dog	85	6.0
Light hot dog	1 hot dog	110	8.4
Veggie dog	1 hot dog	118	7.0
Lean smoked sausage (broiled)	3 oz	120	3.6
Soy/veggie burger	1 patty (about 3 oz)	137	4.1
Burger made from ground top round (broiled, no bun)	3 oz	153	4.2
Burger made from ground sirloin (broiled, no bun)	3 oz	166	6.1

Shopping Smarts

Luckily, you don't have to give up these quick mealtime staples. You just need to be more discerning when choosing them. Here are things to keep in mind at the store.

Burgers. Take a good look at that package of "lean" ground beef. What you really want to know is *how* lean. Regular ground beef is about 73 percent lean (which means 27 percent fat)—a 3-ounce cooked patty has 18 grams of fat. Ground round (85 percent lean) is a little better. But ground sirloin (90 percent) and ground top round (97 percent) are wiser choices. A cooked ground sirloin patty has 6 grams of fat—one-third of what that regular ground beef gives you.

Hot dogs. Your best choices in hot dogs are those with 3 grams or less of fat. Look for the words "reduced-fat," "low-fat," or "fat-free" on the label. Don't think that because it says turkey or chicken on the package, it's automatically low in fat. Regular turkey and chicken dogs can still pack 6 to 9 grams of fat each.

LEAN MENU-MAKERS

The more company that hot dog or hamburger has on your plate, the better. But make sure they're worthwhile accompaniments, like the ones below.

Tomatoes and onions. They're loaded with phytochemicals and vitamins that may cut the risk of cancer and heart disease.

Lettuce. Load up on romaine, green- or red-leaf lettuce, and even fresh spinach leaves.

Cheese. Craving a cheeseburger? Opt for a slice of reduced-fat or fat-free American cheese on top instead of full-fat Colby or Cheddar.

Buns. Look to whole grain hamburger and hot dog buns for a fiber boost.

BEST CEREALS

Cereal	Portion	Calories	Grams of Fat	Grams of Fiber
Bran cereal with extra fiber	½ c	50	0.5	13.3
100% bran	⅓ c	80	0.5	8.0
Instant oatmeal with bran and raisins	1 packet (1.4 oz), prepared	158	1.9	5.5
Unsweetened shredded wheat	2 biscuits	160	0.5	5.0
Raisin bran	1 c	190	1.0	8.0
Nugget-type wheat cereal	½ c	200	1.0	5.0
Wheat bran flakes with dried fruit and nuts	1 c	210	3.0	5.0

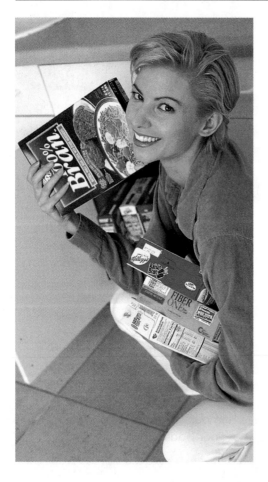

Shopping Smarts

Finding packaged cereals with the least fat and calories—and the most fiber—is easy: Read the ingredient list and Nutrition Facts information on the box. Pay attention to serving sizes: They vary from ½ to 1 cup or more.

Ready-to-eat cereal. Ready-to-eat cold cereal is a calorie bargain—provided you watch out for added sugars in presweetened cereals.

Cooked cereal. Start with the best known—oatmeal, Cream of Wheat, and grits. Then look for other varieties, such as buckwheat, barley, oat bran, or a mixture of whole grains. Quick-cooking and instant varieties save time—just add milk, heat, and eat.

FAT BLASTER

To make the most of cereal, stock your "breakfast center" with other nutrient-rich ingredients such as fresh apples, peaches, pears, apricots, kiwifruit, bananas, berries—whatever fruit you like (to slice or spoon on top).

BEST CHEESES

Cheese	Portion	Calories	Grams of Fat
Fat-free Parmesan cheese	2 tsp	20	0.0
Fat-free cream cheese	1 oz	30	0.0
Fat-free mozzarella	1 oz	35	0.0
Low-fat American processed cheese	1 slice	40	1.0
Fat-free Cheddar cheese	1 oz	45	0.0
Low-fat Cheddar cheese	1 oz	50	1.5
Low-fat mozzarella	1 oz	50	1.5
Reduced-fat feta	1 oz	50	3.0
Fat-free cottage cheese	½ c	90	0.0
Low-fat (1% to 2%) cottage cheese	½ c	90	1.5

Shopping Smarts

Low-fat cheeses are good sources of calcium, so you get this bone-building mineral even while you save fat and calories.

Here's how to select the low-fat cheeses that best meet your needs.

Cheddar, Swiss, and other aged cheeses. You'll find fat-free or reduced-fat versions of some, but not all, types of aged cheese. In general, low-fat cheeses have better cooking qualities than their fat-free counterparts.

Processed cheeses. American cheese, cheese spreads, and other pasteurized blends aren't ripened or aged. As a result, they don't have the same distinct flavor and texture as aged cheese. But they're versatile and keep longer than aged cheese.

Cottage cheese, ricotta, and cream cheese. For the lowest fat and calorie counts, look for fat-free or 1% milk-fat cottage cheese and fat-free cream cheese. Reduced-fat and fat-free ricotta work well in baked dishes, such as lasagna.

FAT BLASTER

In cheese spreads, extend a small amount of stronger-flavored cheese, such as Asiago, blue cheese, feta, sharp Cheddar, or Romano cheese, with fat-free yogurt or cottage cheese.

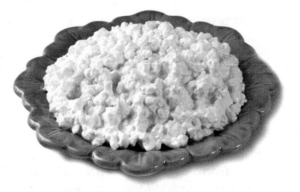

BEST CHICKEN AND POULTRY

Entrée	Portion	Calories	Grams of Fat
Sliced, skinless roasted turkey	3 oz	133	2.7
Barbecued, skinless chicken breast	3 oz, with 2 Tbsp barbecue sauce	167	3.7
Grilled chicken kebabs	2 skewers	170	4.0
Lemon turkey cutlet	1 cutlet, sautéed with lemon and herbs	186	5.3
Oven-fried, skinless chicken	1 leg and thigh, with buttermilk and bread crumb coating	220	8.8
Grilled, skinless chicken breast	½ breast (3 oz), with rosemary and black olives	245	8.0

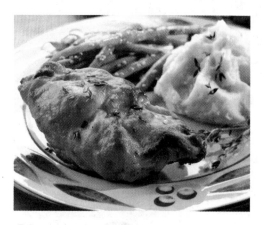

Shopping Smarts

Years ago, buying and cooking poultry was simple: You bought a whole bird then either roasted it or cut it up for other dishes. Today, you can buy chicken part by part, with or without skin, with or without bones, raw or precooked. Here's a look at how to make the best of what's available.

Boneless, skinless chicken breasts and thighs. Cut boneless breast meat into strips, then keep a package or two in your freezer. It will come in handy for stir-fries, fajitas, and chow mein.

Chicken breasts, thighs, or legs, on the bone, with skin. These

LEAN MENU-MAKERS

If chicken and turkey dominate your menus, add variety by trying Rock Cornish game hens, pheasant, and quail. Game hens are available at many supermarkets, and you can ask a butcher to order pheasant or quail. Although they cost more, these low-fat, high-nutrition birds are a unique taste sensation. Three skinless ounces of each (about the size of your palm) has a skimpy 3.3 grams of fat and about 20 grams of protein. And there's no need to seek out exotic recipes for these birds: Game hens, pheasant, and quail can be roasted just as you would a chicken or turkey.

pieces are great for marinating and grilling because they hold in flavor and moisture. If you're going to baste the meat with a sauce such as barbecue sauce, remove the skin first to allow the sauce to cook in and flavor the meat more fully. Otherwise, remove it before eating.

Skinless chicken breasts or thighs on the bone. This type of chicken is best for oven frying or skillet dishes.

Whole chicken. Roasting chickens are meant for roasting, not frying or grilling. The whole bird generally has more fat than individual pieces without skin, so roast it on a rack to allow the fat to run off, and remove the skin before serving.

Turkey breast. Choose the real thing, not the processed version. (Processed turkey is a combination of pressed white and dark meat, and it's loaded with salt.) Roast it covered to lock in the moisture, and enjoy the leftovers on salads and in sandwiches.

Ground turkey. Beware: Regular ground turkey is no leaner than most ground beef, so reach for the extra-lean version. Three ounces of regular ground turkey has more than 11 grams of fat, while the same amount of extra-lean light meat ground turkey has just 2.6 grams.

FAT BLASTER

Keep in mind that chicken and turkey are interchangeable in many recipes. Try these:

• Enjoy extra-lean ground turkey as patties, in chili, and in any recipe for ground beef.

• Grill chicken burgers instead of hamburgers.

• Cook ground turkey or chicken with taco seasoning for a low-fat taco filling.

Real Women SHOW YOU HOW

She Doesn't Go Overboard

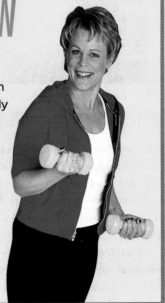

When Sue Torpey, 46, joined a weight-loss program last year, the travel business that she owns was really starting to grow. Unfortunately, so was her waistline. Hosting one food-filled cruise after another, she was really worried about her weight. "The food is unbelievable on these cruises, and it's available 24 hours a day!" she says. "Now I've learned that as long as I stick to lifting weights and eating sensibly at other times, I don't gain weight!"

Because Sue allows for indulgences but doesn't overdo them, she has lost 14 pounds and kept them off.

BEST CONDIMENTS AND SPREADS

Condiment	Portion	Calories	Grams of Fat
Tabasco (hot pepper) sauce	1 tsp	1	0.0
Thick and chunky salsa	1 Tbsp	5	0.0
Prepared horseradish	1 Tbsp	6	0.0
Fat-free mayonnaise	1 Tbsp	10	0.0
Sugar-free jam	1 Tbsp	10	0.0
Yellow mustard	1 Tbsp	12	0.0
Ketchup	1 Tbsp	16	0.0
"Light" tub margarine-like spread	1 Tbsp	35	3.5

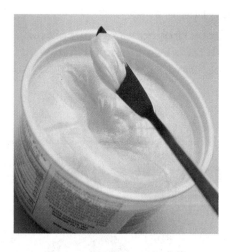

Shopping Smarts

If you've been trying to lose weight, you probably switched to fat-free or reduced-fat mayonnaise and "diet" margarine years ago. Here are a few category-specific tips to help make the most of the zillion choices in the condiments and spreads aisle.

Fat-free or reduced-fat mayonnaises. Good start: Per tablespoon, low-fat (or light) brands contain 50 fewer calories and 6 fewer grams of fat than regular mayonnaise, and fat-free varieties run about 90 fewer calories and 11 fewer grams of fat than regular.

Butters, margarines, and margarine-like spreads. As a table spread, "calorie-reduced" or "light" tub margarine-like spread is your best bet. Try different brands to find the flavor and texture that appeals most to you. Don't use reduced-fat spreads and margarines for cooking, though—they're higher in water, so they won't brown foods, and they can ruin baked goods.

Look for margarine or margarine-like spreads made with olive or canola oils. These products are higher in monounsaturated fats and are less likely to clog coronary arteries than other vegetable oils, which are higher in saturated fat, a factor associated with heart disease. Also, look for varieties that are free of trans fatty acids (by-products of the manufacturing process that make margarine solid at room temperature and affect your heart like saturated fats do).

Mustards. Brown, yellow, smooth, coarse—most contain a scant 4 to 10 calories per teaspoon and virtually no fat. Be adventurous—try Dijon, Parisian, stone-ground varieties, and those with added herbs. For a sweet touch, try honey mustard, but be aware that 1 tablespoon has 30 calories, not 4 or 5. So spread thinly.

Tartar sauces, horseradishes, and relishes. You won't go wrong here—provided you look for low-fat tartar sauce and prepared horseradish, not the cream sauce variety. No luck? Just mix some pickle relish or prepared horseradish with a tablespoon or two of fat-free mayo.

Jams, jellies, and marmalades. Standard fare in most households, fruit spreads are pure sugar—but not off-limits. Substituting 1 teaspoon of jam or marmalade for 1 teaspoon of butter or margarine on breads, bagels, and English muffins cuts calories from your spread by more than half. The key is to buy the best strawberry preserves, orange marmalade, raspberry jam—whatever is your favorite—and then enjoy just a little. Or try fruit butter for a lower-calorie, less sugary alternative.

Bottled sauces. From good old Texas-style barbecue sauce to Oriental duck sauce, you'll find a virtual United Nations of flavor enhancers available for meat, chicken, and fish: steak sauce, teriyaki, miso (a soy product), hoisin, Szechuan—plus the standard soy sauce and ketchup.

Salsas. The Mexican word for "sauce," salsas are cooked or fresh mixtures of tomatoes, sweet peppers, hot peppers, and onions. Traditionally, there were just two salsa staples: "salsa cruda," which was uncooked tomato-based salsa, and "salsa verde," or green salsa made from raw tomatillos, green chile peppers, and cilantro. Today the selection is wider, with varieties that are chunky or spicy, or that use all

---

LEAN MENU-MAKERS

Mix up these flavor-boosting condiments and spreads, serve them on chicken, fish, and veggies, and be bored no longer.

- Pasta sauce with peppers, mushrooms, and garlic
- Salsa with frozen chopped broccoli (proportions to taste)
- 2 tablespoons of mustard mixed with 1 tablespoon of balsamic vinegar
- 2 tablespoons of orange or apricot marmalade mixed with 1 tablespoon of soy sauce
- 1 teaspoon peanut butter, 1 tablespoon soy sauce, and 1 teaspoon each minced garlic and fresh ginger
- Fat-free mayonnaise and freshly chopped rosemary (1 tablespoon each), and one clove garlic, minced

---

kinds of vegetables or even fruit. Most salsas are fat-free, but double-check the label, and bypass any laced with cheese or oil.

FAT BLASTER

A cross between mustard and mayonnaise, mustard-mayo blends give mayonnaise lovers lots of the creamy taste, with just 5 calories and no fat per teaspoon (enough for a sandwich).

BEST DELI FOOD

Deli Item	Portion	Calories	Grams of Fat
Reduced-fat cheese	1 oz	90	7.0
Sliced turkey	3 oz	92	1.3
Sliced ham	3 oz	93	3.0
Sliced roast beef	3 oz	94	2.5
Sliced turkey pastrami	3 oz	120	5.3
Rotisserie chicken breast (without skin)	½ breast	142	3.1
German potato salad	1 c	167	2.2

Shopping Smarts

In a deli, it's easy to be overcome with smells and desires. Keep your wits about you, and don't be afraid to ask questions. Here are some important things to keep in mind.

Meats. Despite their reputation, lunchmeats today are leaner than ever. So a deli sandwich isn't necessarily a bad choice. The lowest-fat lunchmeats are turkey breast, chicken breast, roast beef, turkey pastrami, and—yes!—ham, whether plain or honey-glazed.

Sandwiches. To save calories, consider setting half the meat aside for tomorrow's sandwich. Or order half a sandwich.

Salads. As for side salads, look for ones without a creamy dressing (for instance, choose pickled cabbage instead of creamy coleslaw and three-bean salad rather than macaroni salad).

FAT BLASTER

A pickle may be all you need to satisfy that urge for a crunchy, salty snack to go with your deli sandwich. Pickles are nothing but seasoned cucumbers, so they're completely fat-free and very low in calories.

LEAN MENU-MAKERS

Since the produce department is usually just steps away from the deli in supermarkets, you can easily buy vegetables and fruit to round out your deli choices.

• Bagged salads are convenient complements to sandwiches and rotisserie chicken. Select those without dressing and grab a bottle of low-fat or fat-free dressing while you're in the store.

• Bagged baby carrots and broccoli and cauliflower florets are good raw or steamed. They are an easy way to add nutrient-rich vegetables to a deli meal.

• Broccoli coleslaw is a nice change from regular coleslaw. Buy bags of broccoli slaw and add low-fat coleslaw dressing.

BEST DESSERTS

Dessert	Portion	Calories	Grams of Fat
Poached fruit topped with toasted oatmeal	1 peach and 2 Tbsp oatmeal	55	0.0
Fat-free pudding (prepared from a dry mix with fat-free milk)	½ c	70	0.0
Meringue cookies	4 cookies (about ¾ oz)	73	0.0
Sorbet	½ c	80	0.0
Angel food cake with fresh fruit	1 slice (¹⁄₁₂ of cake)	85	0.0
Biscotti	1 cookie (about ¾ oz)	100	3.0
Low-fat frozen yogurt	½ c	110	2.5
Gingersnaps	4 cookies (about 1 oz total)	120	2.5
Strawberries with low-fat frozen yogurt	¼ c sliced berries with ½ c frozen yogurt	122	2.5

Shopping Smarts

To prepare low-calorie, low-fat desserts from scratch, stock the following staples.

Pantry staples. If you like to bake (or your family expects it), keep the following items on hand.

▶ Whole wheat flour, oatmeal, and other whole grains, such as barley flour (to boost the fiber content in baked goods).

▶ Low-fat or fat-free dairy products for baked dishes. (You can substitute fat-free evaporated milk and buttermilk for cream.)

▶ Naturally sweetened fruit spreads, applesauce, and prune butter (to replace part of the fat in baked goods).

▶ Sugar substitutes. (Read the tips for use on the package. Those with aspartame aren't appropriate for cooked or baked desserts.)

▶ Vegetable oil spray (to coat baking pans).

LEAN MENU-MAKERS

Have a hankering for apple pie? Try these tasty yet helpful-to-your-waistline treats instead.

• Baked apple (a cored apple stuffed with an oatmeal-and-brown-sugar mixture)

• Apple flan (sliced apples topped with orange juice concentrate and slivered almonds and baked just until tender)

• Crisp apple and cheese slices (freshly sliced apples and reduced-fat Cheddar cheese)

BEST EGG AND EGG DISHES

Egg	Portion	Calories	Grams of Fat
Scrambled egg substitute	Equivalent to 1 egg	35	0.0
Poached egg (yolk well-cooked)	1 egg	75	5.0
Hard-cooked egg	1 egg	78	5.3
Egg salad made with fat-free mayonnaise	½ c	98	5.3
Vegetable omelette made with egg substitute	Substitute equivalent to 2 eggs	125	4.0

Shopping Smarts

Basically, you have two choices when buying eggs—whole eggs or egg substitutes. Here's what to use and when.

Whole eggs. Whether the shells are white or brown makes no difference in nutrient or calorie content. Four jumbo eggs equal five large eggs or six small eggs.

Egg substitutes. These are blends of egg whites, fat-free milk, cornstarch, and vegetable oil, plus some vitamins and minerals. They look like raw scrambled eggs, and they have no cholesterol and as little as 35 calories per ¼ cup. Check the Nutrition Facts panel for calorie and nutrient content since some have fat, but others don't.

You'll find egg substitutes in the frozen foods and refrigerated cases in your supermarket. You can use them to replace some or all of the whole eggs or egg yolks in your breakfast or in baked goods.

FAT BLASTER

Prepare a hard-cooked egg instead of a fried egg for breakfast. To save time in the morning, prepare hard-cooked eggs the night before while dinner is cooking, then refrigerate.

LEAN MENU-MAKERS

Whether you use whole eggs, a combo of whole eggs and egg whites, or egg substitutes, don't let high-calorie accompaniments overshadow their benefits. Here are some serving suggestions for popular egg dishes.

Omelettes or crepes. Fill with stir-fried vegetables, such as spinach, asparagus, peppers, onions, mushrooms, and tomatoes. Or prepare with flaked crabmeat and serve with fresh berries and a whole wheat baguette.

Scrambled eggs. Top with tomato salsa and wrap in a wheat tortilla. Or serve with a sliced tomato and sprouts and layer on a whole wheat English muffin for a breakfast sandwich.

French toast. Make with toasted whole grain bread, and top with sliced kiwifruit and berries and a dollop of thick yogurt.

BEST FAST FOOD

Fast Food	Portion	Calories	Grams of Fat
Soft taco	1 taco	220	10.0
Grilled steak soft taco	1 taco	230	10.0
Baked potato (with ½ cup broccoli and 2 pats of butter)	1 potato	244	8.5
Small hamburger with bun (without condiments)	1 hamburger	260	9.0
Sub sandwich with lean turkey, ham, and vegetables (no mayo)	1 sandwich (6 in)	280	5.0
English muffin sandwich (with egg, Canadian bacon, American cheese, and buttered muffin)	1 sandwich	290	12.0
Grilled chicken sandwich (without mayonnaise)	1 sandwich	370	9.0
Bean burrito	1 burrito	380	12.0

Shopping Smarts

Ask the person at the counter for nutrition information for the food served. Many places either have brochures on hand or post the information on the wall.

Burgers. Think in terms of reasonable portions—kid-size, if necessary. Ask for burgers to be prepared without special sauces or to have the sauce served on the side.

Mexican. Mexican establishments like Taco Bell offer items featuring refried beans, a fiber-filled change from meat. You're better off choosing a bean burrito with 12 grams of fat than a Big Beef Burrito Supreme weighing in at 23 grams of fat.

Chicken and fish. Pay attention to how they're cooked. Are they grilled without extra sauces and toppings? Or are they breaded and fried? There's a huge difference in the amount of fat and calories between the two.

Baked potatoes. Wendy's has baked potatoes—get a plain spud and top it with healthy salad-bar choices like peas, onions,

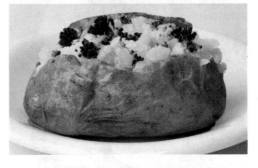

tomatoes, and green peppers. Or order a small bowl of chili to top your spud.

Salads and sandwiches. Subway has a wide variety of salads with fat-free dressings. (Try the roasted chicken breast salad: It has 162 calories and 4 grams of fat.)

FAT BLASTER

Small *anything* is better than supersize or jumbo. A better idea: Go with a side salad and reduced-fat dressing instead of fries. And ask for plenty of tomatoes. They're virtually fat-free.

BEST FISH AND SEAFOOD

Entrée	Portion	Calories	Grams of Fat
Steamed crabmeat	3 oz	87	1.5
Haddock (broiled or baked)	3 oz	95	0.8
Albacore tuna packed in water	3 oz	105	1.5
Steamed shrimp with 2 Tbsp cocktail sauce	3 oz	114	0.9
Tuna (broiled or grilled)	3 oz	118	1.0
Broiled lobster tail with lemon juice	6 oz	166	1.0

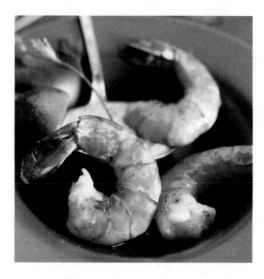

Shopping Smarts

You don't have to go to the best fish market in town every time you want to have fish. These days, your local supermarket has all you need.

Canned fish. Water-packed tuna isn't the only canned fish you can eat when you're trying to watch your calories. Look for water-packed versions of salmon and clams. If you like sardines and anchovies, save them for special occasions.

Frozen fish. Supermarkets compete with fish markets and offer a virtual smorgasbord of fish. In addition to the old standards, you can find just about any finfish that's fit to eat—swordfish, perch, orange roughy, monkfish, snapper, catfish.

Throw a couple of fillets on the grill with some lemon and herbs, and you've added zero fat and calories but a whole lot of zip in just minutes. Or whip up a fish stew or chowder with fat-free milk. Serve with a salad and oyster crackers, and it's chow time.

Imitation fish. Check the frozen fish case for fully cooked, packaged fish labeled as imitation crab, imitation lobster, and imitation scallops. Commonly made from whitefish, they are exceptionally low in fat; in fact, most varieties are fat-free.

Just open a package and top your salad with a generous 3 ounces of imitation crabmeat chunks.

FAT BLASTER

Clam chowders and lobster bisques are made with cream, so if you must indulge, order by the cup, not the bowl—and split it with your dining partner.

BEST FRUIT SELECTIONS

Fruit	Portion	Calories	Grams of Fat
Frozen unsweetened fruit	½ c	26	0.0
Canned fruit packed in juice	½ c	50	0.0
Unsweetened applesauce	½ c	52	0.0
Mixed fruit	½ c	58	0.0
Fresh fruit	1 medium	60	0.0
Fruit juice	¾ c	79	0.0

Shopping Smarts

A generation ago, certain fruits were available only in the summer. While fruit usually is sweeter and more flavorful when it is in season, you can now buy almost any type of fruit all year long.

Fresh fruit. Nothing beats a fresh, crisp apple or a juicy peach. When it comes to fresh fruit, quality is what counts. Look for firm fruit, without bruises or signs of decay.

Canned or frozen fruit. To ensure that you always have some kind of fruit on hand, even when you don't have time to get to the store, stock up on canned and frozen fruit, like applesauce, canned peaches, pears, and pineapple.

Dried fruit. Toss smaller amounts of raisins, dried bananas, cranberries, apricots, and apples into salads, breakfast cereals, pancake batters, and mixed dishes. Dried fruits are nutrient-packed, so by all means, include some in your shopping cart.

Fruit juice and fruit drinks. Check out the Nutrition Facts labels and ingredient lists for 100 percent juice and juice blends. Be aware that fruit-flavored drinks are mainly water and sweeteners.

Fruit bars, spreads, and pastries. Because many of these offer little in the way of fruit and much in the way of calories from added sugar, they don't really count as fruit choices. Opt for the real thing instead.

LEAN MENU-MAKERS

Consider these imaginative ways to eat lean with fruit.

- For breakfast, spread a seasonal array of sliced fruit or berries on a toasted waffle and serve with hot chocolate.

- For lunch, serve mixed fruit in half of a cantaloupe with low-fat or fat-free yogurt and fruit-nut bread.

- Serve a bowl of chilled fruit soup (berry, melon, peach, mango) with a bagel and herbed yogurt cheese.

- For an elegant but light supper, fold mixed fruit into a warm crepe and top with fruit yogurt.

BEST GRAVIES AND SAUCES

Gravy or Sauce	Portion	Calories	Grams of Fat
Tomato sauce	¼ c	18	0.2
Fat-free gravy	¼ c	20	0.0
Au jus gravy	¼ c	24	0.3
Reduced-fat cream of mushroom soup	¼ c	35	1.5
Regular meat gravy	2 Tbsp	40	3.0
Fat-free caramel sauce	2 Tbsp	100	0.0
Cranberry sauce	¼ c	100	0.1
Fat-free chocolate sauce	2 Tbsp	110	0.0

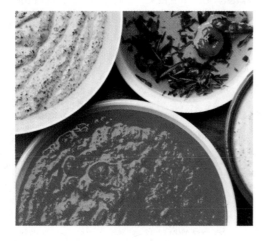

Shopping Smarts

In addition to looking for lighter versions of your sauce favorites, think of entirely new ways to jazz up the plain meat, vegetables, or even dessert on your plate. Then go to the market with these tips in mind.

Gravies. The major manufacturers offer all sorts of fat-free gravies. In addition to regular beef, pork, chicken, and turkey gravy, you'll find mushroom, zesty onion, au jus, slow-roasted types, rotisserie flavors, and more on the supermarket shelf.

Creamy sauces. If it's creaminess that you're after, try reduced-fat condensed soups. Thinned-down cream of chicken, mushroom, celery, and broccoli soups make good toppings for simply prepared chicken, fish, and rice.

Other savory sauces. Make leftover vegetables work for you. Puree cooked red peppers, broccoli, or carrots with broth or wine. Start with 1 cup of vegetables and 1 tablespoon of broth or wine. Add more liquid if you want a thinner sauce or more vegetables if you want a thicker one. Add the seasonings of your choice. The sauce can be used as a topping for meat, poultry, or seafood.

Dessert sauces. Try fat-free chocolate, vanilla, or butterscotch pudding (make it thinner by using an extra ½ cup of milk when you cook it). Or go with flavored yogurt (add a little grated orange rind to kick up the flavor a notch).

FAT BLASTER

Knock off calories in creamy sauces by substituting fat-free evaporated milk for cream.

BEST MEAT SELECTIONS

Meat	Portion	Calories	Grams of Fat
Lean roast beef from deli	3 slices (3 oz)	120	4.5
Canadian bacon	3 slices (3 oz)	129	5.8
Pork tenderloin	3 oz	139	4.1
Roasted beef eye of round	3 oz	141	4.0
Beef top round	3 oz	169	4.3
Flank steak	3 oz	176	8.6
Broiled pork sirloin chops	3 oz	181	8.6
Lamb shish kebabs	3 oz	190	7.5

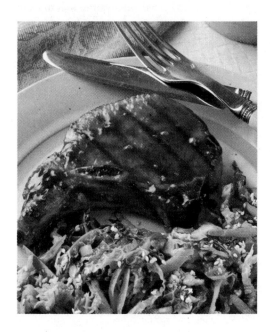

Shopping Smarts

When shopping for meat, think, "Buy less, eat less." Here are some of the best buys at the meat counter.

Beef. Find out whether the beef your market sells is graded prime, choice, or select.

Prime has the most fat marbled throughout; select, the least. Choose cuts with the word *loin* or *round* in the name for the fewest calories and least fat. Eye of round, top round, round tip, top sirloin, bottom round, top loin, and tenderloin are the lowest-fat choices.

Pork. The leanest cuts are tenderloin, sirloin chops, loin roast, top loin chops, loin chops, sirloin roast, rib chops, and rib roast. Check your market for Smithfield Lean Generation Pork, which is specially bred to be low in fat—it's 35 to 61 percent leaner than traditional pork.

Veal. The cuts that are lowest in fat include arm, blade, steak, rib roast, loin chops, and cutlets.

Lamb. Look for arm chops, loin chops, shank, and leg roast. Grill the chops, braise the shank, and make vegetable-rich stew with the leg meat.

FAT BLASTER

Make tacos and burritos with only half the meat. Toss in rinsed canned beans to make up the difference.

BEST MILK AND DAIRY SELECTIONS

Food Item	Portion	Calories	Grams of Fat
Fat-free milk	1 c	85	0.4
Low-fat buttermilk	1 c	99	2.2
Sherbet	½ c	102	1.5
1% milk	1 c	102	2.6
Unsweetened fat-free yogurt	1 c	137	0.4
Soy milk	1 c	141	2.8
Low-fat chocolate milk	1 c	158	2.5

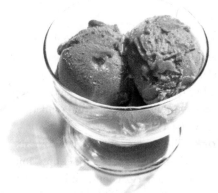

Shopping Smarts

If you're watching your weight, you're probably already buying fat-free or reduced-fat milk. Here are some other things to consider.

Reduced-fat milk. At 4.7 grams of fat and 121 calories per cup, 2% milk (reduced-fat) is a great intermediate step in coming down from whole milk to fat-free. Switching to fat-free (zero gram of fat and 85 calories per cup) can help you shed the pounds that shave off inches effortlessly.

Sour cream. Use reduced-fat sour cream (1.8 grams of fat and 20 calories per tablespoon) or fat-free sour cream (no fat and 13 calories per tablespoon).

Cream cheese. If you're like many people, you may have a hard time making the switch to fat-free, preferring instead the low-fat variety. So compromise: Buy the low-fat and fat-free versions and mix them together, creating a version with 1.4 grams of fat and 25 calories.

Yogurt. To select yogurt, start by homing in on products that are fat-free. Then check out the calories. Choose a product with no more than 120 calories in 8 ounces or 100 calories in 6 ounces. Or look for plain, vanilla, or lemon fat-free yogurt and slice your own fruit into the container.

Frozen yogurt and ice cream. Experiment with flavors that interest you, such as black raspberry swirl fat-free frozen yogurt or caramel-praline crunch fat-free frozen yogurt. Limit your serving to ½ cup, which has less than 150 calories and no fat.

FAT BLASTER

Individual serving–size milk drinks are an easy way to carry fat-free milk to work or on camping trips. If you like your milk cold, refrigerate or pack it on ice before serving.

BEST PASTA AND TOPPINGS

Pasta or Topping	Portion	Calories	Grams of Fat
Parmesan cheese	1 Tbsp	23	1.5
Pasta	1 c cooked	197	1.0
Pasta primavera (with garlic and oil, not a cream-based sauce)	About 3 Tbsp sauce over 1 c cooked pasta	239	4.5
Linguine with red clam sauce	½ c sauce over 1 c cooked pasta	257	2.0
Pasta with clam sauce (water, clams, oil, and spices)	¼ c sauce over 1 c cooked pasta	267	6.0
Pasta with marinara sauce	½ c sauce over 1 c cooked pasta	268	2.6

Shopping Smarts

Happily, you don't have to give pasta the boot when cutting calories. Just keep these things in mind when shopping.

Pasta. With so many shapes and sizes available, you can have pasta every night for weeks without ever repeating a meal. Buy strands like spaghetti and fettuccine, tubes like penne and ziti, various colored spirals, and shells of all sizes.

Check labels carefully when buying fresh pasta, especially stuffed types like ravioli, cappelletti, and tortellini. Fresh pasta often contains eggs and is generally higher in fat than dried. In addition, the fillings in stuffed varieties are usually high in fat.

Sauce. Stick with low-fat meatless tomato sauces rather than creamy ones like Alfredo and pesto. Even reduced-fat pesto can have 4 grams of fat in just 1 tablespoon. Fat content can vary widely among tomato sauces, so check labels.

Pasta-ready tomatoes are also a good choice and are very low in fat. Look for flavors other than Italian for a change of pace. Taco-style Mexican sauce can give your pasta a whole new identity.

Cheese. Buy a thin wedge of really good cheese (like Parmigiano-Reggiano or Pecorino Romano) and grate it at the table.

FAT BLASTER

Mix heated marinara sauce with pureed low-fat cottage cheese. You'll get creaminess and pleasing texture without a lot of calories.

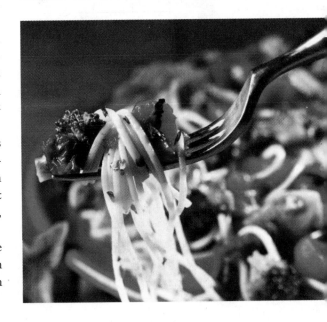

BEST PIZZA AND TOPPINGS

Pizza	Portion	Calories	Grams of Fat
Thin-crust cheese pizza with peppers, mushrooms, and onions (fast-food)	1 slice (⅛ of pie)	190	8.0
Homemade pizza (with low-fat prepared pizza shell, fat-free sauce, 8 oz part-skim mozzarella cheese, and 1 c steamed vegetables)	1 slice (⅙ of pie)	211	3.1
Thin-crust cheese pizza (fast-food)	1 slice (⅛ of pie)	225	10.0
Thin-crust cheese pizza with 1 oz Canadian bacon	1 slice (⅛ of pie)	268	12.0

Shopping Smarts

It pays to purchase healthy pizza ingredients. That way, you can concoct a nutritious and satisfying meal on a moment's notice—and for a lot less than what a pizzeria pie costs (in dollars *and* calories). Here's what to buy.

Crust. Look in the refrigerated case for prepared pizza crust. There are ready-formed

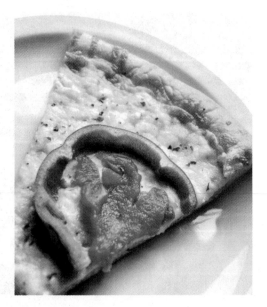

ones and those in a tube. Either way, check labels to find the lowest in fat. Sometimes plain crusts are also available in the freezer section. Don't forget the box mixes; prepare them with less oil than is called for in the recipe.

LEAN MENU-MAKERS

Unless you're careful, pizza tends to be top-heavy with calories and fat. Here are some slimming substitutions.

- Sun-dried tomatoes can stand in for pepperoni. They have a similar look, but the intensely flavored tomatoes are much lower in fat.

- Instead of sausage, try eggplant, portobello mushrooms, broccoli, jalapeño chile peppers, spinach, tomato slices, artichoke hearts, or zucchini.

- Skip the cheese and pile on more vegetables to take up the slack.

Real Women
SHOW YOU HOW

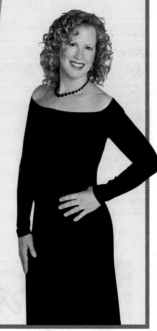

She Lost Weight—with Pizza!

"**I** guess I'll have to give up my pepperoni pizza, huh?" asked Eileen Fehr, 47, when she began her weight-loss program a year ago. Much to her surprise, she didn't. She just had to add fiber-filled fruits and vegetables to her meals. "Now I'm satisfied with less—even when it's a corned beef sandwich or pizza!" she says.

Eating more fiber has also allowed Eileen to forgo calorie counting. Fiber actually whisks some of the calories you eat through your digestive system before they have a chance to settle on your waistline. Now 15 pounds trimmer, Eileen is living proof of fiber's weight-loss powers.

Sauce. There are lots of low-fat pizza and pasta sauces from which to choose. Look for ones with 4 grams or less of fat per ½ cup. Try different flavors to give your pizza extra sparkle.

Cheese. Pick up reduced-fat shredded cheeses. Mozzarella is standard, but it needn't be your only choice. There are good Italian and Mexican cheese blends, for instance, that make terrific pizza. Limit cheese to 8 ounces per large pizza.

Other toppings. Favor veggies like onions, bell peppers, mushrooms, and pickled hot peppers—even a few olives, if you like. Buy super-lean ground beef or ground turkey breast. They're better meat choices than pepperoni, sausage, meatballs, and salami. Brown the ground meat in a nonstick skillet and drain it well before sprinkling it over the crust. Cana-dian bacon and lean ham are good replacements for regular bacon.

Frozen pizza. Steer clear of frozen deep-dish pizza; the fat is out of sight. If you must purchase frozen pizza, pick the thin-crust varieties. Enhance their nutrition by adding steamed or sautéed vegetables, lean ground beef, or diced cooked chicken. (Leftovers work great as pizza toppings.)

FAT BLASTER

For an instant no-fuss pizza, top a sliced English muffin or slice of pita bread with fat-free pizza sauce and 1 ounce of reduced-fat cheese. Heat under the broiler or in a toaster oven until the cheese melts.

BEST SALAD DRESSINGS

Salad Dressing	Portion	Calories	Grams of Fat
Balsamic vinegar	1 Tbsp	10	0.0
Fat-free mayonnaise	1 Tbsp	10	0.0
Fat-free Italian	2 Tbsp	15	0.0
Fat-free French	2 Tbsp	30	0.0
Fat-free vinaigrette	2 Tbsp	35	0.0
Low-fat raspberry vinaigrette	2 Tbsp	35	1.5
Fat-free ranch	2 Tbsp	40	0.0
Low-fat blue cheese	2 Tbsp	40	1.5

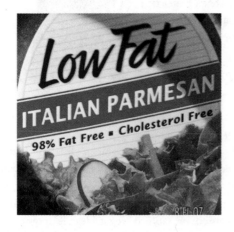

Shopping Smarts

When time is short or if you're all thumbs in the kitchen, the quickest way to put your salad on a diet is to stock up on bottled reduced-fat or fat-free salad dressings. Here's what to look for.

Prepared salad dressings. To find those with the fewest calories, you'll want to check out the Nutrition Facts on the food label, and you'll have to experiment to find which ones you like best.

Vinegars. Vinegar has practically no calories and can be paired with any oil—in proportions you control—plus a number of savory herbs and flavorings. Start with the basics: cider vinegar, red wine vinegar, and white vinegar.

Oils. All oils have about the same amount of fat and calories—14 grams of fat and 125 calories per tablespoon. The difference is the amount of saturated fat, not total fat. Olive oil is high in monounsaturated fat, which can actually help lower your total cholesterol count. Don't assume that "light" olive oil has fewer calories— it's simply lighter in flavor and color, not fat.

Seasonings. To keep your tastebuds stimulated, don't stop with oil and vinegar. Boost the flavor of homemade dressings with fresh herbs. Tarragon, oregano, basil, and parsley are basics.

FAT BLASTER

In place of high-fat dressings, fill a spray bottle with a full-flavored oil to lightly spritz your greens. You'll end up using much less oil.

BEST SNACKS

Snack Food	Portion	Calories	Grams of Fat
Baby carrots with 1 Tbsp fat-free ranch dip	5 carrots	45	0.0
Air-popped popcorn	3 c	90	0.0
Cereal bar	1 bar	92	3.0
Baked tortilla chips	13 chips (1 oz)	110	1.0
Baked potato chips	11 chips (1 oz)	110	1.5
Roasted soy nuts	⅓ c (1 oz)	150	7.0

Shopping Smarts

To find nutrient-dense snacks, read more than just the information about fat and calories on the label. Look for fiber, calcium, iron, and other vitamins and minerals. Here are some noteworthy noshes.

Cereal bars. These tend to be a better choice than granola bars because they're lower in fat and higher in nutrients. What really sets them apart, though, is the fact that cereal bars are fortified with between 10 and 50 percent of your Daily Value for many vitamins and minerals.

String cheese. This mozzarella-like cheese offers a helping of calcium without a lot of fat—as long as you don't eat the whole package. Look for the kind that's portion-controlled in sticks of ¾ ounces.

Nuts. They're filled with fiber, iron, and all kinds of trace minerals and immunity-enhancing nutrients. Their biggest drawback, of course, is fat (even though it's heart-smart unsaturated fat). But if you learn to eat just a handful to satisfy that snack urge, you can reap their nutritional benefits.

Popcorn. Air-popped popcorn has only 30 calories and no fat in 1 cup. Microwave pop-

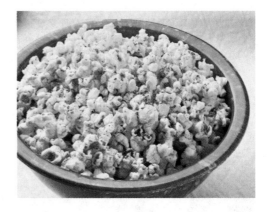

corn is a whole other animal. If you can't resist microwave popcorn, look for light or low-fat types.

Chips. Save half the calories and all the fat by eating fat-free potato chips instead of regular potato chips. Low-fat tortilla chips have 90 calories and 1 gram of fat in a serving, compared with 142 calories and 7.4 grams of fat for regular.

FAT BLASTER

Try Oreo cereal in place of Oreo cookies (it's fortified with extra vitamins and minerals that the cookies don't have).

BEST SOUPS AND CHOWDERS

Soup	Portion	Calories	Grams of Fat
Miso soup	1 c	35	0.0
Gazpacho	1 c	56	0.2
Vegetable soup	1 c	90	2.0
Minestrone	1 c	120	2.0
Bean soup, made without bacon	1 c	130	0.5
Chicken soup, made with defatted broth	1 c	160	3.0

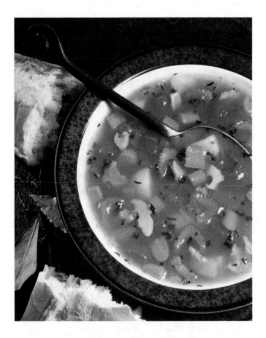

get. Whether you make soup from scratch or buy prepared soups, these health-smart tips can help you stock a soup-ready kitchen.

Canned broth. Stock your pantry with vegetable broth and fat-free beef and chicken broth—they serve as the base for all kinds of flavorful homemade soups.

Ready-to-eat soups or condensed soups. Ready-to-eat soups simply need to be heated. With condensed soups, some of the water is removed, so you need to reconstitute them before heating. For more flavor and nutrients, use milk, broth, vegetable juice, or water left over from cooking vegetables instead of plain water when you heat them.

Dehydrated soups. Most are low in fat. To prepare, just add hot liquid, perhaps low-sodium broth.

Shopping Smarts

To find soups with the least amount of fat and calories, read the Nutrition Facts labels. Clear soups are usually lower in fat and calories than creamy soups. You'll also find low-fat and fat-free versions of cream of mushroom, cream of celery, and other higher-fat soups. Very often, the heartier the soup, the more nutrients you

FAT BLASTER

To lighten up a cream-based soup, replace the cream with a calcium-rich alternative such as fat-free evaporated milk, low-fat buttermilk, or low-fat milk fortified with nonfat dry milk.

BEST TACOS, TORTILLA FILLINGS, AND WRAPS

Item, filling, or topping	Portion	Calories	Grams of Fat
Salsa	2 Tbsp	10	0.0
Fat-free sour cream	2 Tbsp	20	0.0
Corn tortilla	1 tortilla (1 oz)	70	0.6
Fat-free refried beans	½ c	100	0.0
Baked tortilla chips	13 chips (1 oz)	110	1.0
Flour tortilla	1 tortilla (1¼ oz)	115	3.4

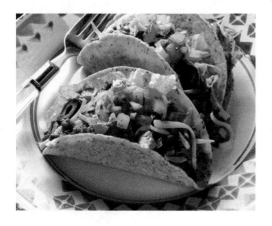

Shopping Smarts

Wrap up quick, nutrition-minded meals today—starting with the tortillas, wraps, fillings, sauces, and seasonings you buy.

Tortillas. You can buy soft wheat and corn tortillas in various sizes, keep them on hand in your refrigerator or freezer, and use them to suit your needs when you and your family are hungry but time for dinner is short.

Fillings. For quick and satisfying tacos, wraps, and other filled tortillas that help you reach your calorie target, stock your kitchen with a variety of these ingredients.

▶ Canned beans. Refried beans are great in burritos; just add salsa. Look for the fat-free varieties. Drained kidney beans, chickpeas, black beans, and other canned beans make great filling "combos" with ground meat or veggies for Mexican dishes or international wraps with Greek, Asian, or Italian ingredients.

▶ Lean ground turkey or lean ground beef, boneless chicken breast, and lean stir-fry beef or pork for your freezer.

▶ Canned crabmeat or tuna. Combined with rice, crabmeat or tuna is great for Asian-style wraps.

▶ Chopped frozen vegetables. Mix them into vegetarian tortilla-wrap fillings, or combine them with meat, chicken, or seafood fillings.

FAT BLASTER

For a hearty main dish or nutritious snack, fill tortillas with a mixture of lean and low-fat ingredients from a variety of sources, focusing on grain products, beans, vegetables, lean meats or dairy, and even fruit. (Helpful hint: Warm the tortillas so they're easier to roll.)

Chapter 3

Fat-Blasting Recipes the Whole Family Will Love

Meals so tasty, no one will know they're good for you!

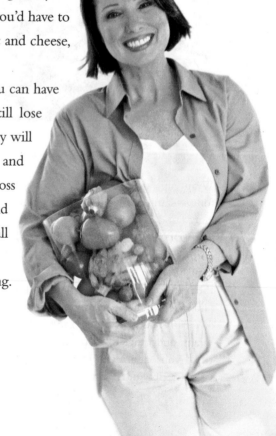

When you set out on this program, you might have thought that you'd have to say goodbye to pizza, mac and cheese, rich gravies, and desserts.

So you'll be thrilled to learn that you can have your beloved homemade dishes and still lose weight. Best of all, this is food your family will love. We've taken familiar family recipes and made them over to meet your weight-loss needs! You still get the same rich taste and the same feeling of comfort—without all the calories and fat.

So put on your apron and get cooking. Eating lean has never tasted this good!

GOOD-FOR-YOUR-WAISTLINE MUFFINS

These muffins are great as an on-the-go breakfast. They have 251 fewer calories than the cupcakelike confections that masquerade as breakfast food. To cut the fat from your own muffin recipes, use two egg whites or ¼ cup of fat-free egg substitute in place of each whole egg. Replace whole milk with fat-free milk, and reduce the oil to 1 tablespoon per cup of flour.

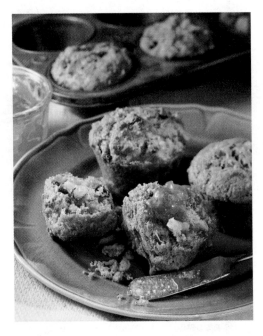

¾ cup unbleached flour

¾ cup whole wheat flour

¼ cup oat bran

1½ teaspoons baking powder

½ teaspoon ground cinnamon

⅛ teaspoon ground allspice

½ teaspoon grated orange peel

¾ cup orange juice

1 egg white, lightly beaten

2 tablespoons canola oil

2 tablespoons honey

1 medium carrot, shredded

Preheat the oven to 400°F. Coat 10 muffin cups with cooking spray (or line the cups with paper baking cups). Set aside.

In a medium bowl, stir together the unbleached flour, whole wheat flour, oat bran, baking powder, cinnamon, and allspice.

In a small bowl, combine the orange peel, orange juice, egg white, oil, and honey. Add to the flour mixture and stir just until combined. Stir in the carrot.

Spoon the batter into the muffin cups,

filling each about three-quarters full. Bake for 20 minutes, or until a toothpick inserted near the center comes out clean. Remove the muffins from the muffin cups. Cool completely on a wire rack.

To store: Individually wrap each muffin in freezer paper or resealable freezer bags and freeze until ready to serve.

To serve: Thaw overnight at room temperature. Or thaw and reheat each muffin in a microwave oven on high power for 15 to 20 seconds.

Makes 10 muffins

Per muffin: 119 calories, 3.2 g fat (23% of calories from fat)

Variation: For a special treat, stir in some raisins.

FAT BLASTER

Let raisins or other dried fruit stand in for all or some of the nuts in quick breads and muffins.

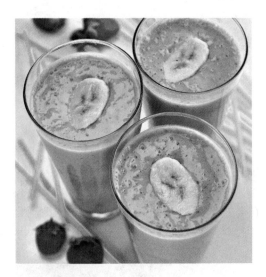

STRAWBERRY-BANANA SMOOTHIE

Made properly, fruit smoothies make an excellent breakfast drink or midday pick-me-up. In contrast, the bottled versions are sticky sweet with fruit syrup, and you'll get stuck with lots of extra calories—often in excess of 300 calories per 8 ounces—and with very little nutrition to show for the calorie burst.

2 cups frozen sliced strawberries

1 large banana, sliced

½ cup orange juice

½ cup fat-free vanilla yogurt or fat-free milk

6 ice cubes

In a blender, combine the strawberries, banana, orange juice, yogurt or milk, and ice cubes. Blend until thick and smooth.

Makes 4 servings

Per serving: 85 calories, 0.5 g fat (5% of calories from fat)

Real Women SHOW YOU HOW

She Tricked Her Tastebuds

Linda Snyder does not like to experiment with new foods. But by making over her favorite recipes, she found that she could eat what she liked and still pare off 11 pounds. For instance, by removing the skin from chicken legs and thighs, dipping them in buttermilk and herbed bread crumbs, spritzing them with cooking spray, then baking them, Linda gets fried chicken flavor but with 200 fewer calories and over 20 fewer grams of fat per serving. There are plenty of low-fat and low-cal cookbooks available to help you learn how to make over your favorites, too.

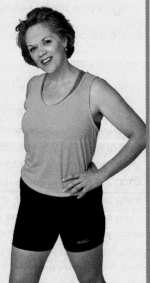

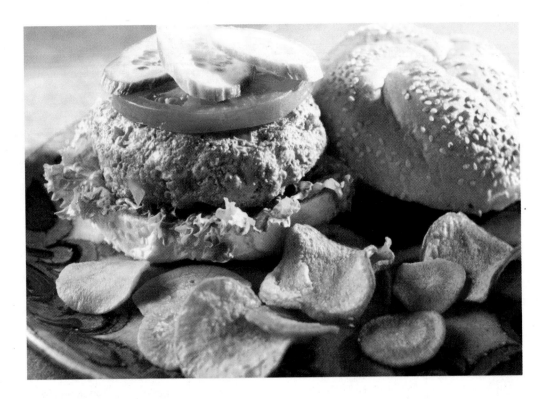

CALIFORNIA-STYLE TURKEY BURGERS

One of these tasty burgers has 13.4 fewer grams of fat than a same-size burger made of ground round. To make the leanest patties possible, purchase boneless, skinless turkey breast. Cut it into chunks and grind it in a food processor using on/off turns. If you're serving fewer than 12, you can freeze the extra turkey mixture for future quick patties. Just form the patties, stack them (separated with pieces of waxed paper), wrap well, and freeze.

3 pounds ground turkey breast

1 cup minced onion

1 cup celery

1 cup minced red bell pepper

¼ cup tomato paste

2 cloves garlic, minced

1 teaspoon ground black pepper

12 crusty rolls

Shredded lettuce

Tomato slices

In a large bowl, thoroughly mix the turkey, onion, celery, red pepper, tomato paste, garlic, and black pepper.

Form into 12 patties. Grill (or broil or sauté in a nonstick skillet).

Serve in the rolls with the lettuce and tomatoes.

Makes 12 servings

Per burger: 289 calories, 2.6 g fat (8% of calories from fat)

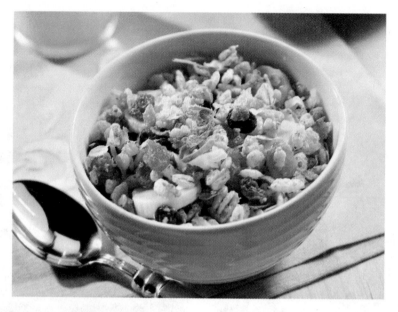

THREE-GRAIN GRANOLA

Despite its reputation for being healthy, granola—especially the commercial variety—is often alarmingly high in fat and calories. It can contain as much as 8.6 grams of fat and 225 calories per ½-cup serving. Toasting the grains and adding honey help to make up for not using any added fat.

2 cups puffed rice

1⅓ cups bran flakes

½ cup old-fashioned rolled oats

¼ cup raisins

2 tablespoons toasted wheat germ

½ cup unsweetened apple juice

2 tablespoons honey

Preheat the oven to 300°F. In a medium bowl, combine the puffed rice, bran flakes, oats, raisins, and wheat germ.

In a small bowl, stir together the apple juice and honey. Pour over the puffed rice mixture and toss until moistened.

Coat a 15" × 10" baking pan with cooking spray. Spread the puffed rice mixture in the pan. Bake for 30 minutes or until golden brown, stirring twice during baking.

Transfer the granola to a large piece of aluminum foil. Let the mixture cool, then break it into pieces.

To store: Transfer the granola to a container. Cover loosely and store at room temperature until ready to serve. (Do not cover tightly because the cereal will not stay crisp.)

To serve: For each serving, place ¾ cup granola in a cereal bowl and add ½ cup fat-free milk.

Note: If you want to splurge a little, stir ¼ cup flaked coconut into the cereal mixture before baking. You'll get an extra 35 calories and 2.4 grams of fat in each serving.

Makes 4 servings

Per serving: 250 calories, 1.5 g fat, (5% of calories from fat), 3.5 g of fiber

BAKED MACARONI AND CHEESE

This stripped-down version of the American classic has 153 fewer calories and 24 fewer grams of fat than a standard version. For even more flavor, sprinkle a little grated fat-free Parmesan cheese on top, along with herbs such as minced parsley. To make over your family's favorite cheese dish, use a reduced-fat Cheddar (or blend a strong-flavored, full-fat sharp Cheddar cheese 50-50 with a reduced-fat variety) and replace butter and whole milk with more reduced-fat cheese and fat-free milk.

    8   ounces elbow macaroni

    1   tablespoon olive oil

    1   tablespoon all-purpose flour

    ½   teaspoon mustard powder

    1¼ cups fat-free milk

    1¼ cups shredded low-fat extra-sharp
        Cheddar cheese

    ½   cup light ricotta cheese

    2   tablespoons chopped scallions

        Salt

        Ground black pepper

    ¼   cup toasted bread crumbs

Preheat the oven to 375°F. Coat an 8" × 8" baking pan with cooking spray. Set aside.

Cook the macaroni according to the package directions. Drain well.

Meanwhile, heat the oil in a 3-quart non-stick saucepan over low heat; stir in the flour and mustard. Cook and stir for 1 minute.

Gradually stir in the milk. Bring to a boil; cook and stir for 1 minute. Add the Cheddar. Remove the pan from the heat.

In a blender or food processor, puree the ricotta. Add to the sauce. Stir in the scallions and pasta; add salt and pepper to taste. Spoon into the baking pan. Top with the bread crumbs. Bake for 20 minutes, or until the top is golden brown.

Makes 4 servings

Per serving: 415 calories, 10.8 g fat (24% of calories from fat)

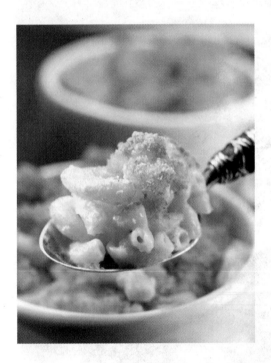

OVEN-FRIED CHICKEN

The simple step of switching to "oven frying" makes this all-American favorite healthier. This version has 5.4 fewer grams of fat than the equivalent serving of a fried chicken thigh. To trim calories and fat from your other favorite chicken recipes, remove the skin and use egg whites instead of melted butter to make coatings stick.

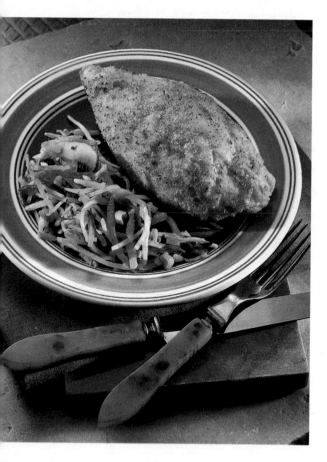

½ cup buttermilk

1 cup fresh bread crumbs

1 teaspoon paprika

1 teaspoon ground black pepper

½ teaspoon dried thyme

½ teaspoon onion powder

4 pieces skinless chicken legs and thighs

Preheat the oven to 425°F. Coat a wire rack with cooking spray. Place the rack on a foil-lined baking sheet.

Pour the buttermilk in a shallow pan. Put the bread crumbs in another shallow pan. Combine the paprika, pepper, thyme, and onion powder in a bowl. Season the bread crumbs with 1 teaspoon of the spice mixture. Add the remaining spices to the buttermilk.

Coat the chicken with the buttermilk. Roll the chicken pieces in the seasoned bread crumbs.

Place the chicken on the prepared rack. Coat the chicken with cooking spray.

Bake for 15 minutes. Turn the chicken, coat it again with cooking spray, and bake for 15 minutes more, or until golden brown.

Makes 4 servings

Per serving: 229 calories, 8.8 g fat (36% of calories from fat)

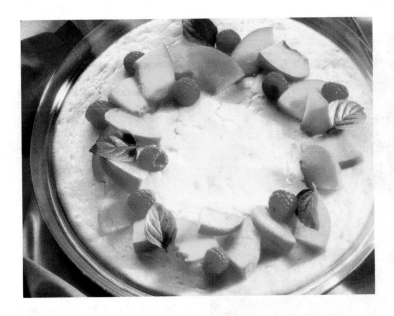

NEW YORK CHEESECAKE

Cheesecake that's low in fat? You bet! Light cream cheese, low-fat ricotta cheese, and a fat-sparse cookie crust reduce the fat without reducing a forkful of flavor. (If you don't have amaretti crumbs, substitute graham crackers.) To make over your favorite cheesecake recipe, substitute light, reduced-fat, or fat-free cream cheese for full-fat cream cheese; fold in stiffly beaten egg whites to add volume; use a dusting of crumbs on the bottom of the pan as a crust; and top with fruit instead of a syrup fruit topping.

8 ounces light cream cheese

1 cup low-fat ricotta cheese

2 eggs, separated

¼ cup honey

¼ cup golden raisins

3 tablespoons cornstarch

1 tablespoon grated orange rind

⅓ cup amaretti cookie crumbs

Preheat the oven to 400°F. In a large bowl, combine the cream cheese and ricotta until smooth. Stir in the egg yolks, honey, raisins, cornstarch, and orange rind, mixing until thoroughly combined.

In a medium bowl, whip the egg whites with clean beaters for about 2 minutes, or until they form stiff peaks. Fold the whites into the cheese mixture.

Coat a 9" pie plate with cooking spray and cover with the amaretti crumbs. Pour the cheese mixture into the pie plate. Bake for 30 minutes, or until golden and set.

Makes 12 servings

Per serving: 121 calories, 5.2 g fat (37% of calories from fat)

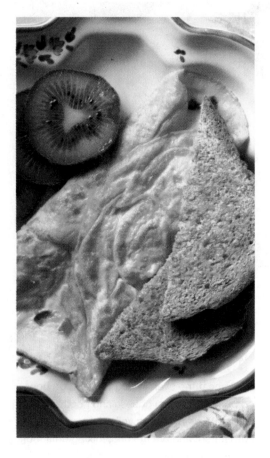

1 cup sliced mushrooms

¾ cup fat-free egg substitute

1 tablespoon water

½ teaspoon dried basil

¼ teaspoon ground black pepper

1 teaspoon margarine

1 tablespoon grated Parmesan cheese

Place the mushrooms in a 2-cup glass measure and cover with vented plastic wrap. Microwave on high for 2 minutes, or until the mushrooms are wilted. Drain off any liquid.

In a medium bowl, whisk together the egg substitute, water, basil, and pepper.

In a medium nonstick skillet over medium heat, melt the margarine. Swirl the pan to coat the bottom. Add the egg mixture. As the eggs begin to set, pull the outer edges toward the center with a fork or spatula; allow uncooked portions to run underneath. Continue until the eggs are just barely set.

Sprinkle with the mushrooms and Parmesan. Fold the omelette in half. Transfer to a serving plate.

Note: If you don't have a microwave, cook the mushrooms in a little bit of fat-free broth until they soften and give up their natural juices. Then cook a few minutes longer to evaporate the liquid.

Makes 1 serving

Per serving: 158 calories, 6 g fat (34% of calories from fat)

BASIL AND MUSHROOM OMELETTE

Parmesan cheese and basil add a lot of flavor to this slimmed-down omelette. You could also make an omelette substituting egg whites for whole eggs and using other vegetables and herbs of your choice (such as broccoli and thyme).

TUNA NOODLE CASSEROLE

This time-honored favorite may not be glamorous, but it can save the day on weeknights when you haven't had time to shop for groceries but don't want to give in to a fast-food meal out of desperation. Round out this one-dish supper with stewed tomatoes—a great source of heart-healthy lycopene—or a satisfying salad of dark leafy greens, green peppers, beans, and other nutrient-dense veggies.

8   ounces no-yolk or whole wheat noodles

1   package (16 ounces) frozen broccoli florets, thawed

1   can (12 ounces) water-packed white tuna, drained and flaked

1   can (10¾ ounces) fat-free, reduced-sodium condensed cream of mushroom soup

1   cup 1% milk

1   cup shredded reduced-fat Monterey Jack cheese

8   ounces fat-free plain yogurt

½   teaspoon ground black pepper

¼   teaspoon celery seeds

¼   teaspoon crushed red-pepper flakes

½   cup crushed reduced-fat snack crackers

¼   cup grated Parmesan cheese

Preheat the oven to 350°F. Coat a 13" × 9" baking dish with cooking spray.

Cook the noodles in a large pot of boiling water according to the package directions. Drain and return to the pot. Remove from the heat; toss with the broccoli and tuna.

In a large bowl, mix the soup, milk, Monterey Jack, yogurt, black pepper, celery seeds, and red-pepper flakes. Pour over the noodle mixture and stir carefully. Transfer to the baking dish.

Mix the crackers and Parmesan; sprinkle over the casserole. Bake for 30 minutes or until lightly browned.

Makes 4 servings

Per serving: 583 calories, 12.8 g fat (20% of calories from fat)

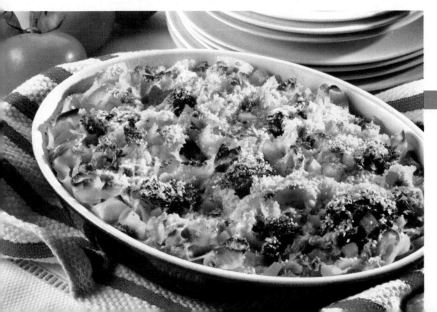

FAT BLASTER

Prepare low-calorie sauces for casseroles by thickening fat-free broth or fat-free milk with cornstarch or arrowroot.

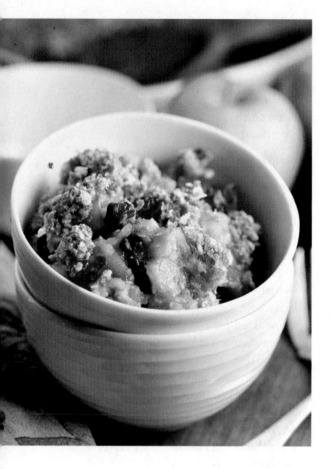

¾ cup old-fashioned rolled oats

⅓ cup whole wheat flour

¼ cup packed dark brown sugar

⅛ teaspoon salt

⅛ teaspoon ground allspice

3 tablespoons chilled unsalted butter or margarine, cut into small pieces

3 large Empire, Idared, or Granny Smith apples, cored and sliced into ¼"-thick wedges

½ cup dried cranberries

3 tablespoons frozen apple juice concentrate

1 tablespoon sugar

Preheat the oven to 425°F.

In a medium bowl, combine the oats, flour, brown sugar, salt, and allspice. Using your fingers or a pastry blender, lightly mix in the butter or margarine until the mixture is crumbly.

In an 8" or 9" square baking dish, toss together the apples, cranberries, apple juice concentrate, and sugar until well-mixed. Sprinkle the oat mixture evenly over the top.

Cover with foil and bake for 20 minutes, or until the mixture is bubbly and the apples are tender. Uncover and bake for 5 to 10 minutes longer, or until the topping is lightly browned.

Makes 8 servings

Per serving: 186 calories, 5.2 g fat (25% of calories from fat)

APPLE-CRANBERRY CRISP

Instead of viewing dessert as a sinful indulgence, consider it an opportunity to reach your daily quota for fruit. This appetizing meal finale focuses on fresh fruit, oats, whole wheat flour, and apple juice concentrate, with a minimal amount of fat and sugar. If you can't get dried cranberries, substitute other dried fruit, such as chopped prunes or apricots.

THIGH-FRIENDLY MUSHROOM GRAVY

If the guys in your household insist on gravy with their turkey and mashed potatoes, you can all ladle up without wrecking your weight-friendly eating plan. This velvety stand-in for giblet gravy will save you 46 calories and 6 grams of fat.

½ cup sliced celery

½ cup chopped carrot

½ cup chopped onion

3 cloves garlic, minced

   Pinch of dried sage

   Pinch of dried thyme

2 cans (14 ounces each) fat-free, reduced-sodium chicken broth

1 package (0.35 ounces) dried mushrooms (found in produce section)

¼ cup all-purpose flour

¼ teaspoon hot-pepper sauce

½ cup fat-free, reduced-sodium chicken broth (optional)

Coat a large nonstick saucepan with cooking spray. Add the celery, carrot, onion, garlic, sage, and thyme. Coat with cooking spray. Cover; cook over medium heat, stirring occasionally, for 10 minutes.

Add the broth and mushrooms. Cover; simmer for 30 minutes. Using a slotted spoon, remove the mushrooms. Chop finely.

Pour the gravy mixture into a blender and add the flour. Puree. Return to the pan, and add the hot-pepper sauce and mushrooms. Reheat to a boil. Add extra broth, if desired, to thin.

Makes 8 servings

Per ½-cup serving: 33.5 calories, 0.1 g fat (3% of calories from fat)

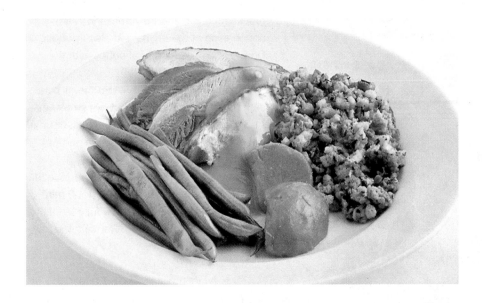

BANISH-THE-FAT BEEF STEW

When it comes to beef, a little bit goes a long way toward helping you reach your shape-up goals, especially when it comes "packaged" with tons of soul-satisfying potatoes and vegetables. You probably have most of these ingredients on hand. If not, you can always substitute, for example, regular onions for the pearl onions.

- 4 small red potatoes, each cut into 6 wedges
- 1 medium turnip, peeled and cut into chunks
- 1 medium parsnip, peeled and cut into chunks
- 1 cup frozen peeled pearl onions
- 3 medium carrots, peeled and cut into chunks
- 1 cup drained canned tomatoes
- 1¾ cups defatted, reduced-sodium beef broth
- 1 tablespoon red wine vinegar
- 2 cloves garlic, crushed
- 1 bay leaf
- ½ teaspoon dried thyme
- ½ teaspoon freshly ground black pepper
- 12 ounces lean, trimmed beef top round or sirloin, cut into ½" cubes
- 1 tablespoon all-purpose flour
- 1 tablespoon olive oil

In a large, heavy saucepan, combine the potatoes, turnip, parsnip, onions, carrots, tomatoes, broth, vinegar, half of the garlic, the bay leaf, ¼ teaspoon of the thyme, and ¼ teaspoon of the pepper. Break up the tomatoes with the edge of a spoon. Cover and bring to a boil over high heat. Reduce the heat to medium and simmer for 25 minutes, or until the vegetables are just tender.

Meanwhile, toss the beef cubes with the remaining garlic and the remaining ¼ teaspoon each of the thyme and black pepper. Dredge the seasoned beef cubes with the flour.

In a large, heavy skillet, warm the oil over high heat until it's very hot but not smoking. Add the beef and sauté for 5 minutes, or until the beef is browned on the outside and medium-rare on the inside.

Add the beef to the vegetables, reduce the heat to medium-low, and simmer for 5 minutes, or until the vegetables are fully tender and the flavors are blended. Remove the bay leaf before serving.

Makes 4 servings

Per serving: 335 calories, 6.9 g fat (18% of calories from fat)

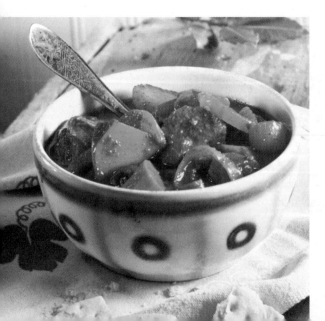

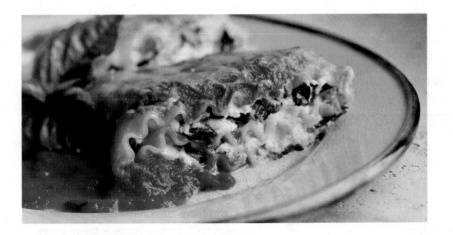

BEEF AND SPINACH LASAGNA

A typical slab of lasagna can easily run you as much as 24 grams of fat. With this slimmed-down version, you can serve the whole family while you stick to your eating-lean plan.

  2 cups reduced-fat ricotta cheese

  1 package (10 ounces) frozen chopped spinach, thawed and squeezed dry

  ½ teaspoon ground black pepper

  ½ teaspoon ground nutmeg

  1 pound lean ground beef top round

  1 teaspoon crushed red-pepper flakes

  ⅛ teaspoon salt

  1 jar (26 ounces) fat-free tomato-basil sauce

  1 box (8 ounces) no-boil lasagna noodles

  5 leaves fresh sage, coarsely chopped

  1 cup shredded fat-free mozzarella cheese

  1 plum tomato, thinly sliced

  5 large leaves fresh basil

  ¼ cup grated Romano cheese

Preheat the oven to 375°F. Coat a 9" × 9" baking dish with cooking spray.

In a medium bowl, combine the ricotta, spinach, black pepper, and nutmeg. Mix well.

Place a large nonstick skillet over medium heat until hot. Crumble the beef into the skillet. Cook, stirring to break up the meat, for 4 to 6 minutes, or until the meat is no longer pink. Drain off any accumulated fat. Add the red-pepper flakes and salt to the beef. Mix well.

Spread ½ cup of sauce in the prepared baking dish. Place 3 or 4 of the lasagna noodles on the sauce so their edges don't overlap. Top with half of the remaining tomato sauce and all of the beef. Sprinkle with half of the sage. Top with another layer of noodles. Spread the ricotta mixture over the noodles and sprinkle with ½ cup of the mozzarella.

Top with a third layer of noodles and the remaining tomato sauce. Top with the tomato, basil, and the remaining sage. Sprinkle evenly with the Romano and the remaining ½ cup of mozzarella.

Cover tightly with foil and bake for 20 to 25 minutes, or until bubbling and heated through.

Makes 4 servings

Per serving: 595 calories, 12.5 g fat (19% of calories from fat)

VEGETABLE PIZZA WITH GOAT CHEESE

Faster than pizza delivery, this homemade pie is in the oven in 10 minutes if you use precut vegetables, prepared pizza dough, and prepared sauce.

1 teaspoon cornmeal

1 pound reduced-sodium fresh pizza dough

2 tablespoons prepared pesto

1 red onion, thinly sliced

1 large tomato, sliced

1 jar (7 ounces) roasted sweet red peppers, drained

1 cup chopped broccoli florets

⅓ cup crumbled goat cheese

2 tablespoons grated Parmesan cheese

Preheat the oven to 500°F. Set the oven rack at its lowest position.

Sprinkle the cornmeal on a large ungreased baking sheet. Roll out the pizza dough and place it on the baking sheet, pressing to fit.

Spread the pesto on the crust. Top with the onion and tomato. Sprinkle the peppers, broccoli, goat cheese, and Parmesan on top. Bake for 10 to 15 minutes, or until the underside is browned and the cheese has melted. Cut into wedges.

Makes 4 servings

Per serving: 375 calories, 10.1 g fat (24% of calories from fat)

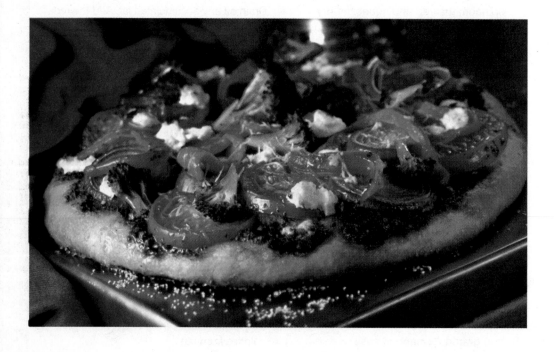

BUTTERMILK MASHED POTATOES

This slimmed-down version of mashed potatoes will satisfy the staunchest meat-and-potatoes fan at your house. Compared to mashed potatoes made with butter and whole milk, you save 127 calories and 8.4 grams of fat per serving.

1 pound (about 3 medium) baking potatoes, such as russets, peeled and cut into 1-inch chunks

1 cup water

½ cup defatted chicken broth

2 garlic cloves, unpeeled

¼ cup low-fat buttermilk

2 tablespoons thinly sliced scallions

⅛ teaspoon freshly ground pepper, preferably white

   Large pinch of salt

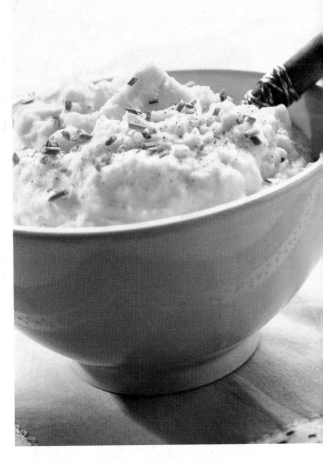

In a medium saucepan, combine the potatoes, water, broth, and garlic. Cover and bring to a boil over high heat. Reduce the heat to medium-low and simmer for 12 to 15 minutes, or until the potatoes are fork-tender.

Just before the potatoes are done, place the buttermilk in a small, heavy saucepan and warm it over low heat.

Drain the potatoes well; discard the garlic cloves. Return the potatoes to the pan and mash them with a potato masher or in a food processor.

Stir the warmed buttermilk, scallions, pepper, and salt into the potatoes and serve.

Makes 4 servings

Per serving: 96 calories, 0.5 g fat (5% of calories from fat)

Real Women SHOW YOU HOW

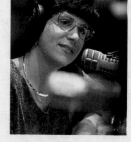

Her Meals Had Makeovers

Teresa Tomeo grew up in a traditional Italian family that loves to eat. Her secret to losing weight? She learned to make slimmer versions of her favorite dishes. She reduced the amount of olive oil in her tomato sauce to a drizzle, and she took out the meat completely and replaced it with veggies. She used vegetable purees to thicken sauces and soups. She topped salads with a squeeze of lemon juice instead of dressing. As a result, Teresa went from 190 pounds to 130, a weight she's maintained for 14 years.

CREAMY BLUE CHEESE DRESSING

A lot of women think that blue cheese dressing is off-limits when they're trying to lose weight. Au contraire! Blue cheese is so flavorful that by pairing a small amount with fat-free cottage cheese, you can save 144 calories and 16 grams of fat. To make over other creamy dressings, substitute pureed fat-free cottage cheese or yogurt for sour cream or other high-fat ingredients and flavor with garlic and herbs.

- 1 cup fat-free cottage cheese
- 2 tablespoons crumbled blue cheese
- 2 tablespoons fat-free milk
- 1 clove garlic, minced

In a blender or food processor, blend or process the cottage cheese, blue cheese, milk, and garlic on low speed for 20 seconds. (The blue cheese will still be chunky.) To store, cover tightly and refrigerate for up to 1 week.

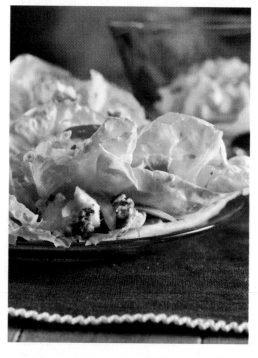

Makes 8 servings or 1 cup
Per 2 tablespoons: 26 calories, 1 g fat (37% of calories from fat)

CHEWY OATMEAL COOKIES

If your gang is clamoring for homemade cookies, you can indulge them (and yourself) without guilt. If you like, substitute ⅓ cup miniature semisweet chocolate chips for ⅓ cup of the raisins. The calories and fat per cookie will increase slightly to 81 calories and 2.1 grams of fat.

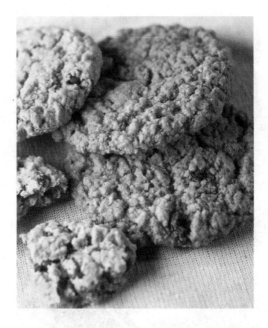

1½ cups all-purpose flour

1 teaspoon ground cinnamon

¾ teaspoon baking soda

¼ teaspoon salt

¼ cup margarine or unsalted butter, at room temperature

½ cup sugar

½ cup packed light brown sugar

1 egg

⅓ cup fat-free milk

1 tablespoon light corn syrup

1 teaspoon vanilla

1½ cups quick-cooking rolled oats

⅔ cup raisins

Preheat the oven to 375°F. Coat 2 baking sheets with cooking spray.

In a medium bowl, combine the flour, cinnamon, baking soda, and salt. Mix well.

In a large bowl, combine the margarine or butter, sugar, and brown sugar. Using an electric mixer, beat on medium speed until blended. Add the egg and beat for 2 to 3 minutes, or until light and fluffy. Add the milk, corn syrup, and vanilla. Beat until blended.

Reduce the speed to low and gradually add the flour mixture, beating until just combined. Stir in the oats and raisins.

Drop the dough by level tablespoons onto the prepared baking sheets. Bake 1 sheet at a time for 8 to 10 minutes, or until lightly browned. Transfer the cookies to a wire rack to cool.

Makes 36 cookies

Per cookie: 76 calories, 1.7 g fat (20% of calories from fat)

FAT BLASTER

Cut back on the amount of sugar you use in recipes. For every ½ cup you eliminate, you save 387 calories. Add a smidgen of cinnamon, nutmeg, or vanilla extract to add sweetness.

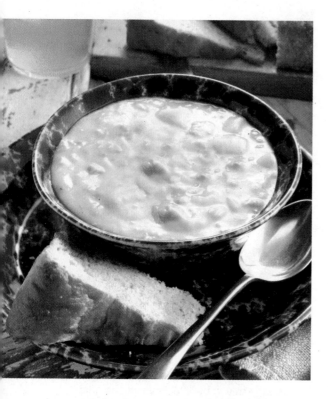

HEARTY SEAFOOD CHOWDER

Thanks to the use of defatted chicken stock and fat-free evaporated milk, this authentic-tasting seafood chowder graces you with nearly 9 fewer grams of fat per serving than conventional chowder made with butter and cream.

12 shucked chowder clams

5 cups defatted chicken stock

2 large baking potatoes, peeled and diced

1 large onion, diced

1 carrot, diced

1 rib celery, diced

1 tablespoon minced fresh parsley

1 bay leaf

½ teaspoon dried oregano

¼ teaspoon dried tarragon

¼ teaspoon ground black pepper

8 ounces cod, cut into 1" pieces

1 cup fat-free evaporated milk

In a 3-quart saucepan, combine the clams and 2 cups of the stock. Bring to a boil over high heat. Reduce the heat to medium and simmer for 3 minutes. Remove the clams with a slotted spoon and set aside.

Add the potatoes, onion, carrot, celery, parsley, bay leaf, oregano, tarragon, pepper, and remaining 3 cups of stock to the saucepan. Bring to a boil, then cook over medium heat for 15 minutes, or until the vegetables are softened. Remove and discard the bay leaf.

Ladle about half of the vegetables and about 1 cup of the liquid into a blender. Blend until smooth. Return to the saucepan. Add the cod and simmer for 5 minutes, or until the cod is cooked through.

Chop the clams finely and add to the saucepan. Stir in the milk and heat briefly.

Makes 4 servings

Per serving: 252 calories, 4.1 g fat (15% of calories from fat)

CHICKEN QUESADILLAS

To enhance the color and flavor of these quesadillas, sprinkle them with an assortment of condiments, such as chopped red bell peppers, onions, tomatoes, and radishes. Altogether, this trimmed-down version of a Mexican favorite has 504 fewer calories and 55 fewer grams of fat than a taco salad.

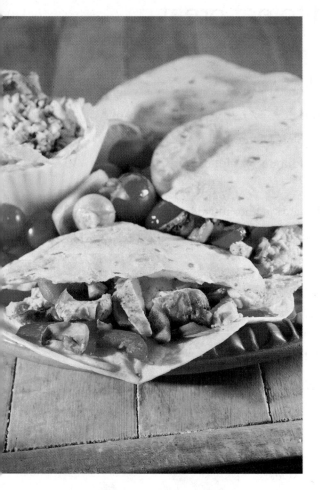

¼ cup lime juice

2 tablespoons chopped cilantro

1 serrano chile pepper, seeded and finely chopped (wear rubber gloves when handling)

4 boneless, skinless chicken breast halves (4 ounces each)

1 red bell pepper, seeded and thinly sliced

1 green bell pepper, seeded and thinly sliced

1 cup scallions sliced into 1" lengths

1 cup thinly sliced mushrooms

½ cup jalapeño jelly

8 flour tortillas, 8" in diameter

Preheat the oven to 400°F. In a shallow bowl, combine the lime juice, cilantro, chile pepper, and chicken. Cover and marinate for 15 minutes. Remove the chicken from the marinade and cook for 6 to 8 minutes over a charcoal fire or in a stovetop skillet, turning once, or until the chicken is cooked through. Thinly slice the chicken on a diagonal.

Coat a large nonstick skillet with cooking spray. Add the red pepper, green pepper, scallions, and mushrooms and cook over medium heat until the scallions are golden and the vegetables are tender. Add the jalapeño jelly and cook until the jelly melts.

Coat a baking sheet with cooking spray. Combine the chicken with the vegetables. Divide among the tortillas. Place the tortillas on the prepared baking sheet and bake for 5 minutes.

Makes 4 servings

Per serving: 401 calories, 5.7 g fat (13% of calories from fat)

Chapter 4

The 7-Day Quick-Start Menu

Everything you need to eat great and lose weight.

We all know what the hardest part of eating to lose weight is: getting started. But now even that part is easy, thanks to our 7-Day Quick-Start Menu. Follow this meal plan, and you'll be well on your way to a thinner, healthier you with hardly any effort!

Designed by Kim Galeaz, R.D., a food and nutrition consultant in Indianapolis, this menu offers three tasty meals a day, plus snacks, for about 25 percent of total calories from fat or less per day.

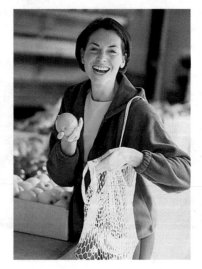

"This meal plan supplies lots of flavor and variety (so you don't get bored) and fiber (so you feel satisfied and full, and don't overeat)," explains Galeaz. "It also keeps you fueled all day long, to maintain energy as you exercise regularly to lose weight and tone up. There's even plenty of room for extras, such as fats, sweets, and treats."

With this menu, you can start banishing your belly, butt, and thighs today by perking up classic family recipes and introducing exciting new foods into your menu. Break out of the rut of eating the same breakfast morning after morning, packing the same three lunch meals week in and week out, or cooking the same four family recipes over and over. Then use what you've learned to expand your weekly menu, using shopping, meal planning, and cooking strategies for eating lean.

"Have fun with flavors and foods," says Galeaz. "Be creative and adventurous."

MONDAY

Breakfast

¾ cup Three-Grain Granola (see page 38) with ½ cup fat-free milk

1 cup fresh grapefruit juice

Snack

1 banana

Lunch

½ whole wheat pita pocket stuffed with 1 ounce lean deli honey ham

6 slices Fuji apple

1 ounce reduced-fat sharp Cheddar cheese, sliced

1 teaspoon light mayonnaise

1 cup green and red pepper strips

Snack

1 Chewy Oatmeal Cookie (see page 51)

1 cup fat-free milk

Dinner

1½ cups angel hair pasta topped with 1 cup commercial pasta sauce

1 cup steamed zucchini and summer squash

1 soft breadstick

Snack

1 cup fat-free white chocolate raspberry yogurt

DAILY TALLY
1,625 calories
20 g fat
11% of calories from fat

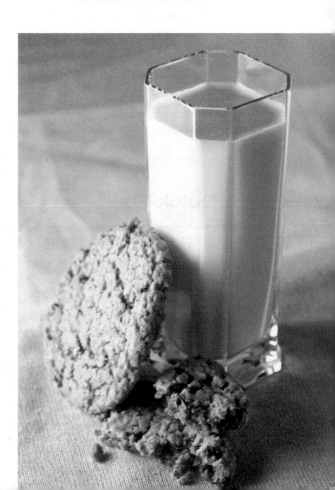

TUESDAY

Breakfast

1 cup vanilla fortified soy milk mixed with 1 packet mocha instant breakfast powder

½ blueberry bagel

1 tablespoon light cream cheese

Snack

1 tangelo

Lunch

California-Style Turkey Burger on crusty roll (see page 37) with shredded lettuce and 2 slices tomato

1 cup broccoli coleslaw mixed with 2 tablespoons low-fat coleslaw dressing

Snack

1 fresh pear

¼ cup roasted, salted soy nuts

Dinner

1 bowl Hearty Seafood Chowder (see page 52)

3 ounces orange roughy, broiled with lemon juice and oregano

1 cup bow-tie pasta

1 cup steamed fresh asparagus spears

Snack

1 cup low-fat chocolate milk

DAILY TALLY
1,652 calories
32 g fat
17% of calories from fat

Real Women SHOW YOU HOW

A Quick Fix

With a full-time career and a 5-year-old son, Brooke Myers, 31, can't afford to spend a lot of time thinking about food. Until recently, that meant using more convenience foods and gaining a few pounds. "We were snacking on lots of junk foods because they were quick and convenient," she says. But the convenience problem was easy to remedy. "Now I stock my kitchen with quick foods that are also healthy," she says. After just 3 weeks of her eating change and exercise, Brooke dropped 11 pounds and lost nearly 3 inches off her waist, 1 inch off her hips, and ¾ inch off her thighs.

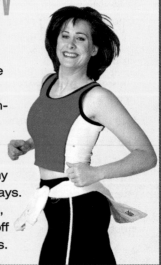

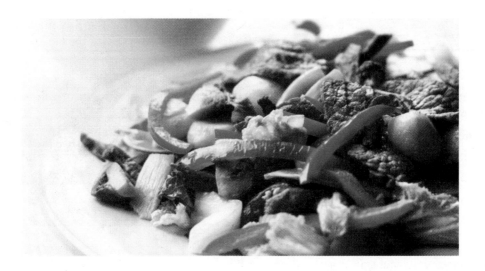

WEDNESDAY

Breakfast

1 fast-food English muffin–and–egg sandwich

1 cup fat-free milk

Snack

1 cup vegetable juice

4 whole grain crackers

Lunch

Deli sandwich made with 2 slices hearty multigrain bread, 1 ounce reduced-fat Swiss cheese, 1 ounce reduced-fat Cheddar cheese, ¼ cup alfalfa sprouts, and 1 teaspoon spicy mustard

Tossed green salad made with 1 cup fresh spinach leaves, ½ cup romaine lettuce, and 1 tablespoon chopped walnuts, and topped with a sprinkling of balsamic vinegar and a squeeze of fresh lemon

¾ cup chopped fresh mango cubes

Snack

¼ cup low-fat spinach dip with 1 mini pita bread, cut into wedges

Dinner

Beef stir-fry made with 3 ounces lean sirloin steak strips and 1 cup Chinese stir-fry vegetables

1 cup brown rice

1 fortune cookie

1 cup honeydew melon cubes

Snack

1 slice New York Cheesecake (see page 41)

DAILY TALLY
1,618 calories
44 g fat
24% of calories from fat

THURSDAY

Breakfast

1 cup fat-free lemon yogurt mixed with 1 tablespoon wheat germ

1 cup fresh strawberries, sliced

Snack

1 Good-for-Your-Waistline Muffin (see page 35)

Lunch

One 3-ounce veggie burger on poppyseed kaiser roll with ¼ cup fresh spinach leaves and 2 slices tomato

12 baby carrots

1 cup fat-free milk

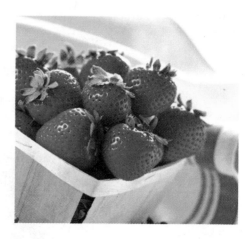

Snack

1 cup black bean soup

4 whole grain crackers

Dinner

1 serving Oven-Fried Chicken (see page 40)

1 serving Buttermilk Mashed Potatoes (see page 49)

1 cup fresh broccoli spears, steamed

1 whole wheat dinner roll

Snack

1 cup fresh red grapes

DAILY TALLY
1,640 calories
26 g fat
14% of calories from fat

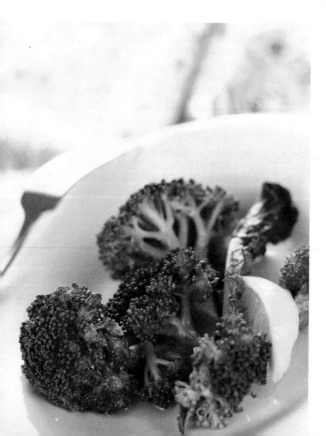

FAT BLASTER

Want to bring out vegetable flavor without adding fat? Steam them. Cook only till crisp-tender, then add seasonings such as herbs, spices, or garlic.

FRIDAY

Breakfast

2 slices cinnamon swirl bread, toasted and topped with 1 tablespoon peanut butter

1 cup cantaloupe chunks

Snack

1 cup low-fat chocolate milk

Lunch

3 ounces albacore tuna, water packed and drained, served over 2 cups mixed fresh spinach leaves, arugula, and red-leaf lettuce, with ¼ cup sun-dried tomatoes

1 serving Creamy Blue Cheese Dressing (see page 50)

1 cup fresh pineapple slices

Snack

4 chocolate graham cracker squares

1 cup fat-free milk

Dinner

1 serving Vegetable Pizza with Goat Cheese (see page 48)

2 soft breadsticks dipped in ½ cup low-fat marinara sauce

Snack

½ cup low-fat strawberry frozen yogurt drizzled with 1 teaspoon chocolate syrup

DAILY TALLY
1,774 calories
36 g fat
18% of calories from fat

Real Women SHOW YOU HOW

She Spiced Up Her Life

By her late thirties, Alice Layne had reached 235 pounds. Her breaking point came when she ordered several outfits for a trip, only to discover in the hotel room that nothing fit. Her group leader at Weight Watchers suggested that she jazz up her menus with international foods. She tried tabbouleh, couscous, and polenta, and she experimented with salsas and spices. She had so much fun trying new foods that she never felt like she was dieting—and her adventurous approach to eating helped her lose 67 pounds and four sizes in just 2 years.

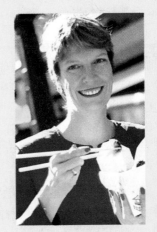

Break out of the weight-loss rut of eating the same food every day. Eating to lose weight can be **adventurous— and easy!**

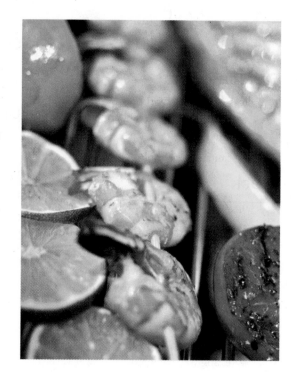

SATURDAY

Breakfast

1 Basil and Mushroom Omelette (see page 42)

1 wheat English muffin

1 teaspoon light margarine

1 cup fresh orange juice

Snack

1 cup fat-free Key lime yogurt

Lunch

3 ounces broiled shrimp kebabs made with ½ a carrot and ¼ of a bell pepper

1½ cups red peppers and zucchini slices, roasted on the grill

½ cup couscous

Snack

1 cup fat-free milk

1 kiwifruit

Dinner

1 serving Chicken Quesadillas (see page 53)

14 baked tortilla chips

¼ cup hot salsa

Snack

½ cup fresh raspberries

2 fat-free mint creme cookies

DAILY TALLY
1,621 calories
27 g fat
15% of calories from fat

SUNDAY

Breakfast

1 sesame seed bagel, toasted and topped with 1 tablespoon apple butter

1 cup fat-free milk

Snack

½ cup fresh blueberries

1 piece string cheese (¾ ounce)

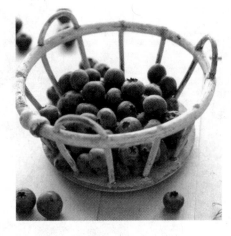

Lunch

1 serving Beef and Spinach Lasagna (see page 47)

1½ cups tossed spinach leaves and romaine lettuce with 4 cherry tomatoes and 2 tablespoons fat-free Italian dressing

1 slice Italian bread sprayed with olive oil vegetable spray and a sprinkling of garlic powder

Snack

¼ cup dried cherries

Dinner

3 ounces lean boneless pork loin (baked, broiled, or grilled) served with Thigh-Friendly Mushroom Gravy (see page 45)

1 baked sweet potato, sprinkled with cinnamon

½ cup steamed fresh green beans

1 whole wheat dinner roll

Snack

6 ounces light cranberry juice cocktail

DAILY TALLY
1,650 calories
27 g fat
15% of calories from fat

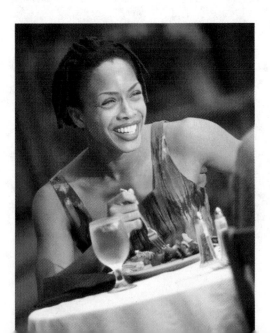

Great news:
You have to eat
to lose weight!

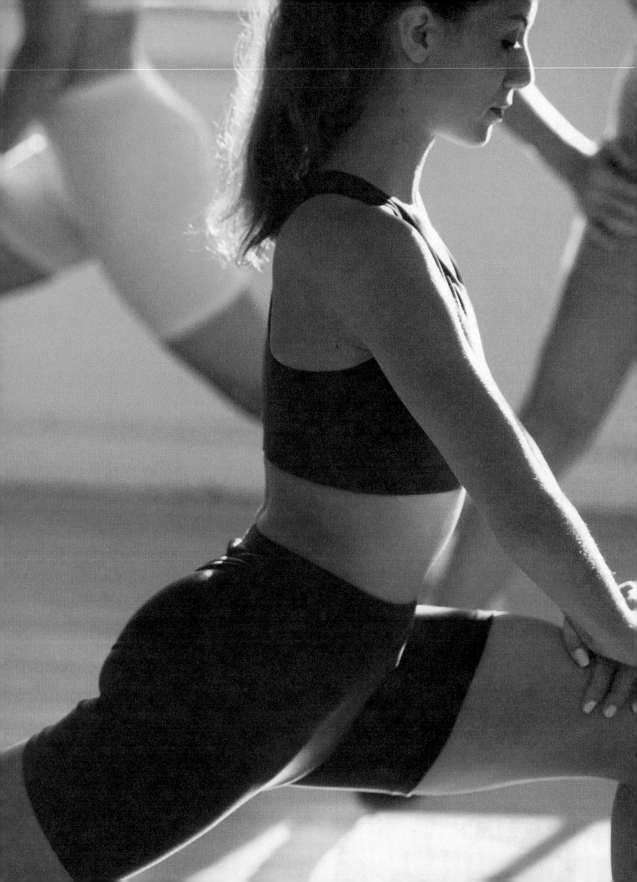

Part 2

The 30-Day Shape-Up Plan

Chapter 5

26 Fun Ways to Work Off Fat and Calories

Skiing, dancing, swimming, even gardening—have fun while you shape up!

You'll be happy to learn that working out aerobically doesn't mean that you have to run or join an aerobics class to lose weight and shape up—unless you want to. Everyday activities like walking and gardening count. They can and do burn fat and calories just like more strenuous workouts and can help women like you flatten their abs, trim their thighs, and tuck their butts.

Aerobic activities are big calorie burners, and—along with a diet that controls fat and calories—they go a long way toward melting away fat. That's because causing your heart to pump at a faster, sustained rate will increase your metabolism during the exercise, burning more calories. It may eventually increase your metabolic rate, the rate at which you burn calories as you go about your daily business. Metabolic changes, in turn, improve your body's ability to burn fat and make your muscles better able to use oxygen for this purpose. As your level of aerobic fitness increases, your heart, lungs, and muscles become more efficient, so you can do more without getting tired.

Once you become more physically active, people may start noticing that you look leaner and more muscular. Most aerobic activity doesn't build muscle, but your muscles will look more toned, and you'll lose fat, so you'll look leaner. For that reason, you'll probably notice that your clothes fit better before you actually see your weight change on the scale.

How Hard Do You Have to Work?

Experts say that to reap all the benefits of aerobic exercise, you need to work at moderate intensity to raise your heart rate for at least 30 minutes a day, three to five times a week.

If you're aiming to lose weight, you need to exercise aerobically at a moderate intensity for 30 to 60 minutes most days of the week. "Thirty minutes is the point at which fat is being used as the primary energy source," says Laurie L. Tis, Ph.D., associate professor in the department of kinesiology and health at Georgia State University in Atlanta.

As you continue to get in shape, what used to be strenuous becomes easier, so you must add to the duration, intensity, or frequency of the exercise, or start doing a different, more challenging activity, says Michael Youssouf, a certified trainer and manager of trainer education and advancement at the Sports Center at Chelsea Piers in New York City. For each of the aerobic activities described in the pages that follow, experts have prescribed beginner, inter-

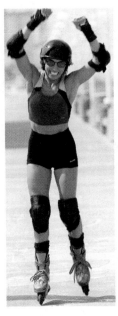

mediate, and experienced levels to help you get started and progress. These levels are not just for safety; they have a built-in success ratio, explains Youssouf. Assign yourself 20 to 30 minutes a day, and make your workout part of your daily routine. Find a level that you can do, and if you enjoy it, you'll keep at it. When you're ready to move on to the next stage, you will.

To banish your belly, butt, and thighs, you can choose from more than two dozen types of activities, from walking or gardening to vacuuming or yard work, described in the pages that follow.

Getting Started

Before you start an aerobic exercise program, ask your doctor for advice if you answer yes to two or more of the following:

▶ You are over the age of 45.

▶ You are younger than 55 and past menopause and not taking estrogen-replacement therapy (which protects your heart).

▶ You smoke cigarettes.

▶ You have or have ever had high blood pressure or high cholesterol.

▶ You're sedentary—that is, you work at a desk, have no physically active hobbies or pastimes, or don't currently exercise regularly.

▶ You have a family history of heart disease, high blood pressure, or high cholesterol.

Calories burned are based on a 150-pound woman. If you weigh more, you'll burn more calories; if you weigh less, you'll burn fewer.

AEROBICS CLASSES AND VIDEOTAPES

Calories Burned

228 per half-hour

Body-Shaping Potential

Tones abdominals, hips, thighs, buttocks, and depending on type of aerobics performed, also other major muscles

Doing aerobics on a regular basis contributes to weight loss and body toning in several ways.

▶ You'll burn fat more efficiently.

▶ You'll tone muscles from head to toe, improving your appearance, strength, and stamina.

▶ You'll improve your flexibility, which extends your range of motion and improves muscle performance, balance, and coordination.

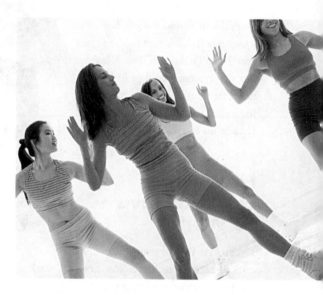

On Your Feet

Shop for cross-trainer shoes, which provide good cushioning, support, flexibility, and traction for performing the variety of exercises that aerobics workouts entail, advise experts at the American Council on Exercise (ACE). If you have high-arched feet, look for a shoe with added shock absorption and more ankle support. If your feet tend to be more flat, look for less cushioning and greater support and heel control.

For a proper fit, allow ½ inch between the end of your longest toe and the end of the shoe. Your shoe should also be as wide as possible across the forefoot without allowing your heel to slip. A well-fitted shoe does require a breaking-in period. If your feet are blistering after a few days, take the shoes back. Finally, replace your shoes regularly. They lose their cushioning after

3 to 6 months of regular use, making you more susceptible to knee and ankle injuries.

Other Stuff You'll Need

Aside from a good pair of shoes, you'll need clothing suited to working up a sweat. And if you'll be exercising on your own, you'll need aerobics videotapes.

Clothes. Look for "breathable" fabrics in a blend of cotton and synthetic fibers that whisk sweat away from your body, allowing you to keep cool.

If the temperature in your workout area varies, wear clothes in a couple of layers that you can take off or put back on as needed.

Videotapes. Aerobics videotapes are a great way to exercise at home—you get to

Real Women
SHOW YOU HOW

Jana Lost 40 Pounds—And Has Kept It Off

When Jana Trabert's family moved to the United States from Korea when she was 12, her introduction to this new world included junk food, TV, and weight gain.

"The American lifestyle is so sedentary," says the 33-year-old interior designer. "Even though I'd been thin in Korea, by my freshman year in high school here, I weighed 150 pounds, and I'm only 5 feet 2 inches tall. I felt fat, yucky, and totally self-conscious."

It was in college when a friend suggested that Jana take an aerobics dance class with her at a local YMCA. She was hooked immediately.

"It was fun," Jana says. "And I started noticing a difference in my body, both on the scale and in the way I looked and felt, after just a couple of months." Working out three times a week, she shed 40 pounds and has kept it off.

While Jana has kept up with her aerobics regimen for about 15 years, these days she does her workouts at home, having traded crowded gyms for her family room, where she plugs in her favorite aerobics exercise videotapes.

"I try to set a certain day and time to do it," Jana says, "but sometimes I get busy—especially since becoming a mother—and I have to just fit it in. And I do. It's not always easy, but it makes me feel great."

enjoy lively music as you follow the moves of other in-shape exercisers bounding across your TV screen. Tapes are available in a wide range of aerobics styles, from traditional choreographed floor aerobics to workouts that help tone specific muscle groups.

Consider the following when choosing a videotape.

▶ **Type.** Look for a workout and music that sparks your personal interest.

▶ **Time.** Figure out realistically how long your workout will be. If your time is limited, use 30-minute videos and put a couple of them together at those times when you can do a longer workout. If you're a beginner, decrease the time or the intensity of your routine if it feels too difficult.

▶ **Intensity.** Don't overestimate what you can do, or you risk getting discouraged right off the bat, says Dr. Tis. You're probably a beginner if you haven't even taken a walk in at least 6 months or you're very overweight. If you walk or do some other form of exercise at least two or three times per week, start as an intermediate.

Getting Started

Here's what you need to get started and keep going with an aerobics exercise program.

Learn the basics. Many aerobics exercises require a degree of motor skill and coordination, which could take time to develop. Start with an introductory class or videotape workout described as low-impact or no-impact, advises Lauri Reimer, director of aerobic instructor training for the Aerobics and Fitness Association of America. As you get comfortable with the exercise program, gradually move into a more advanced workout.

Warm up. Prepare your body and mind for exercise with a 5- to 10-minute warmup of the muscles you will use during your workout, advise experts. Warming up helps your body burn calories more efficiently by increasing your core body temperature. It also helps your muscles work faster and more forcefully, improves muscle elasticity and muscle control, and prevents the buildup of pain-provoking lactic acid in the blood.

Monitor your intensity level. The talk test is a good, commonsense way to judge whether you're working out at a safe pace, says Richard Cotton, chief exercise physiologist for ACE in San Diego. You should be able to carry on a conversation at the same time you're exercising. If you can't, slow down.

Aim for 30 to 60 minutes. Make it your goal to exercise for at least 30 minutes— either at a single stretch or accumulated throughout the day, say experts. If you're an absolute beginner, start out doing only 10 to 15 minutes during the aerobics portion at a low- to moderate-intensity level.

Cool down. As few as 3 minutes of moderate movement like walking after a workout enables your heart and muscles to slowly return to their normal state, says Dr. Tis. Gentle movements and stretches may also help increase or maintain your flexibility and minimize muscle soreness.

FAT BLASTER

Droves of women experienced at aerobics who want to power their workouts have found the answer: martial arts–inspired aerobic workouts like Tae-Bo with Billy Blanks, and Karate Integrated (KI) Aerobics, among others. Experts say that you can figure on burning roughly 280 calories per half-hour— about the same as any intense aerobics class. To find a martial arts-type aerobics class in your area, call your local gym or fitness center. And by the way, experts emphasize that kickboxing-type aerobic routines are geared to intermediate or experienced exercisers, not beginners.

Aerobics Workouts

Beginner	Intermediate	Experienced
10 to 20 minutes, 3 days a week; target heart rate 60 to 65 percent of maximum	20 to 30 minutes, 3 to 5 days a week; target heart rate 65 to 75 percent of maximum	Minimum 20 to 30 minutes, 3 to 5 days a week; target heart rate 75 to 90 percent of maximum

BICYCLING

Calories Burned
130 to 345 per half-hour, depending on the speed and terrain

Body-Shaping Potential
Strengthens and tones all muscles of the lower body, including the butt, thighs, and calves

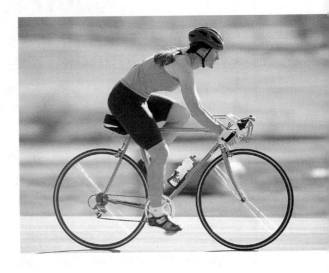

"The body-shaping benefits of cycling are primarily from the hips down," says Edmund Burke, Ph.D., professor of exercise science at the University of Colorado in Colorado Springs and coauthor of *Fitness Cycling*. "Bicycling works the muscles in your buttocks, front and back thighs, and lower legs." So if you bicycle regularly:

▶ You'll strengthen and tone the muscles of your lower body during your workout.

▶ You'll burn off a fair amount of stored calories—or fat.

On Your Feet

Unless you're competing in the world-famous, multi-day Tour de France bike race, you can cycle in comfortable, lightweight sneakers, as long as the soles have enough grip to stay put on the bike pedals, says Dr. Burke.

"Be sure to tuck the laces under the tongue of your shoe, though, so the laces don't get tangled in the pedals, chain, or chain guard," he adds.

Also, don't tie your laces too tightly, or your feet will fall asleep while you ride. To keep your feet comfortable, choose socks made of blends of cotton and synthetic fibers like polypropylene, which wick moisture away and let your skin breathe.

Other Stuff You'll Need

Aside from the right footwear, you'll need a bike and a helmet—both of which you should purchase at a bike shop, where they sell and service bikes. Even if you have an old Schwinn that you want to resurrect, you need to take it over to a bike shop for a tune-up before you head out down the driveway. It's almost sure to need new tires and some oil to lubricate the chains and gears.

If you need a bike, you can choose from three types.

▶ Road bike. This bike looks like a 10-speed, which you may have ridden as a teenager. It has drop handlebars (they curve under) and smooth, narrow tires. These bikes are designed for speed, not comfort.

▶ Mountain bike. These bikes have flat handlebars (they don't curve) and fatter tires than road bikes. It's easier to balance on them. The tires are knobby for better traction. They're designed for riding on unpaved trails, over rocks and roots and

Real Women
SHOW YOU HOW

Saturday Bike Rides Helped Lynn Lose 26 Pounds

Like many women, Lynn Hoerle, 43, found that some of life's rites of passage, such as turning 30, starting a new relationship, and moving to the suburbs, brought something else into her life—weight gain.

"At 5 feet 7, I had always weighed about 125 pounds," says Lynn. "But in my thirties, I found myself weighing 156. I struggled with the extra weight, but I was too busy with work to do anything about it."

Lynn, an office manager, did buy a mountain bike at one point, but it sat in her garage for 3 years, unused. "Then my mother and brother died within a few months of each other," Lynn says. "I realized then that there was more to life than just going to work, so I promised myself I would get out more."

One thing Lynn did was sign up for a 6-week mountain-biking class being held on Saturdays at the local community college. "I learned a lot about biking, but I also learned a lot about Mount Tamalpais, a recreation area where a lot of Northern Californians go to bike and hike," she says. With regular bicycling, Lynn noticed a change in her body shape. "My legs were definitely leaner and stronger," she says. She then followed a structured weight-loss program that included healthier meals. "I basically cut out the junk. No more double chocolate chunk ice cream, no more hunks of cheese after dinner, no more bags of chips."

Lynn now weighs 130 pounds and combines road-racing trips with her mountain-biking outings. "Sometimes, I'm one of the oldest women on the group rides," she says. "Riding motivates me to become fitter, so I can keep up with my friends." She's so motivated, in fact, that for the first time, she recently put on a bathing suit and joined her friends in the hot tub after a long ride. "They'd never seen me in a bathing suit before," Lynn says. "And I felt great, because I didn't feel like an outsider anymore."

such—but they function well on paved paths, too.

▶ Hybrid bike. These bikes have gears, handlebars, and frames similar to mountain bikes but with narrower tires for the smooth ride of a road bike. Experts tend to recommend hybrid bikes for adult women interested in bicycling.

"Hybrids generally have sturdier frames than road bikes, so they provide lots of stability," says Tim Blumenthal, executive director of the International Mountain Bicycling Association in Boulder, Colorado. "They're easy to ride on pavement. And if you want to ride in parks, hybrids can handle dirt trails and unpaved roads."

The right fit. Experts at bike shops are better equipped than salespeople at a department store to measure you and your new equipment properly. Ask for a bike designed especially for women. These have a steeper seat tube (the vertical tube) to position you correctly and a shorter top tube (running from the seat tube to the head tube and handlebars) to accommodate women's shorter torsos and arms. Or they may steer you toward a man's bike that the specialists reconfigure to fit you (moving handlebars or changing the seat, for instance, so you don't have to reach as far for the handlebars). Proper fit is essential. "If your bike doesn't fit you properly, it will be too uncomfortable for you to ride regularly," says Dr. Burke. If you're not experienced at riding a bike with multiple gears, you may want to consider a bike with gears that are clearly numbered, to help you learn how to shift.

A comfortable seat. If you're serious about getting in shape, you'll be spending a fair amount of time in the saddle. So whichever style of bike you choose, you also need to feel comfortable in the saddle.

"You have to find a good bike with a comfortable seat, or else you'll be putting pressure on parts of your body that don't respond well to intense friction and excess weight," says Dr. Burke. So by all means, ask about special seats made for women. Some feature a wider back and narrower, cut-out nose that takes the weight off delicate tissues for a more comfortable ride. Others use a soft material on the underside with less bracing (used for stiffness) than seats for men's bikes, so that the saddle flexes to absorb impact.

A helmet. When you cycle outdoors, you must always wear a helmet to protect your head from impact if you collide with the pavement (or anything else). Many helmets are specially designed for women—a big help if, for example, you want to pull your hair back in a ponytail when you ride. Helmets sold in bike shops are almost always of equal quality because all are made to the same safety specifications. Further, the Consumer Product Safety Commission requires all helmets made or sold in the United States to meet federal safety standards. Consider a helmet with a vent to help keep you cool, and those with reflective stripes and removable visors for riding at night and in the sun. Plan to wear a cap under your helmet only if the helmet is designed to accommodate a hat—otherwise, you compromise fit and safety.

Bicycling Workouts

Beginner	Intermediate	Experienced
Cycle nonstop for 20 minutes on flat terrain, two or three times a week for 3 to 4 weeks.	Beginning on flat terrain, cycle fast for 20 to 30 minutes, then include a couple of hills or shift to a harder gear for 5 minutes at a time, without necessarily going fast. Do this three times a week until you work your way up to riding comfortably 60 minutes each time.	Extend one of your regularly scheduled rides, probably on the weekend, to at least 1½ to double the time or distance of a weekday ride. Vary the speed and intensity as you ride: Climb hills, ride quickly for a few minutes, and use more intensity at other times.

CROSS-COUNTRY SKIING

Calories Burned

486 to 1,116 per hour, depending on the speed and terrain

Body-Shaping Potential

Tones the abdomen, buttocks, hips, thighs, calves, arms, shoulders, and upper and lower back

Cross-country skiers get a tremendous allover workout. Here's what you can expect if you decide to glide, according to Christopher Proctor, M.D., a physician for the U.S. Ski Team and an orthopedic surgeon in Santa Barbara, California.

▶ You'll tone your entire body as you strengthen the major muscles in your feet, legs, buttocks, abdomen, back, arms, and shoulders.

▶ You'll improve your chances of permanent weight loss, because cross-country skiing is one of the best ways to burn calories and fat.

▶ You'll get a fabulous aerobic workout and improve your cardiovascular fitness.

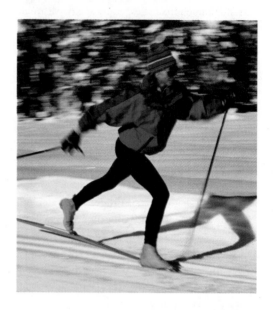

On Your Feet

In cross-country skiing, choosing the right footwear is just as important as choosing the right skis. A knowledgeable salesperson at a reputable ski shop can get you properly outfitted. Here's what you'll need, says Carole Lowe, ski instructor and co-owner with her husband of Rendezvous Ski Tours in the Grand Teton Mountains near Jackson Hole, Wyoming.

Boots. Expert cross-country skiers usually invest in ultralight boots that resemble tennis shoes, Lowe says. But beginners should stick with classic boots, which look more like hiking boots and provide light ankle support.

Bindings. As their name suggests, the bindings hold the toes of your boots against your skis. They leave your heels free to rise with each step in a normal walking motion. Bindings are standardized to fit certain types of boots. Have the salesperson verify that your bindings and boots are compatible as well as check that your boots and skis are compatible.

Socks. Socks should be warm but not too thick. You can find wool-silk blends of ski socks at ski shops, but the best ski socks are made of high-tech polyester, such as Thorlo brand wick socks, according to Lisa Feinberg Densmore, a former member of the Women's Pro Ski Tour, producer and host of numerous ski fitness videos, and instruction editor for *Mountain Sports and Living* magazine in Hanover, New Hampshire. "The poly variety not only wicks moisture but also inhibits odor. They help keep your feet dry and toasty as you ski," she says.

Real Women
SHOW YOU HOW

Skiing Helped Kim Avoid Midlife Weight Gain

Five years and 25 pounds ago, Kim Neifert turned to cross-country skiing as a way to keep exercising through the winter. "I started out just wanting to avoid midlife weight gain," recalls the 39-year-old teacher of emotionally disturbed teenagers. But she came to relish her peaceful excursions into the snowy countryside near Lehighton, Pennsylvania.

"I almost always go alone or with my dog, Honey," Kim says. "I have a very stressful job. Skiing gives me a chance to get back to nature and clear my head."

Even before she started losing weight, Kim noticed her abdomen, hips, inner thighs, and upper arms becoming firmer. Once she made dietary changes to complement her exercise routine (she also walks year-round and kayaks when weather permits), the pounds began to disappear.

Kim prefers to do her skiing in state parks and on open-space trails—mostly on weekends, in the gathering dusk after school, or on nights made silvery white by a full moon. "I even mark my calendar," she says of her moonlit outings. "I can't begin to describe how beautiful those evenings are."

Other Stuff You'll Need

If you're new to cross-country skiing, consider renting equipment to start. A complete package including skis, poles, boots with bindings, gaiters, and even the trail fee costs $20 to $30 a day—about what you'd pay to rent downhill ski equipment. So for a relatively modest fee, you can go on a few trial runs before deciding if cross-country skiing is for you.

Whether you rent or buy, follow these guidelines when selecting equipment and preparing to hit the cross-country trail.

Skis. Cross-country skis are sometimes called skinny skis—presumably for how they look but arguably for what they can do for your figure. They are lighter and thinner than downhill skis, and they range in length from 180 to 200 centimeters. The pair you choose should be roughly 10 centimeters longer than your height. To check length, stand one ski at your side, then raise your adjacent arm overhead. You should be able to comfortably cup your hand over the end of the ski, says Lowe.

Also, look for skis that are textured on the underside, says Lowe. The grooves provide traction on the snow, eliminating the need for waxing (which serves the same purpose).

Poles. Cross-country poles are designed to propel the skier forward. This is why they are longer than downhill poles. Beginning cross-country skiers should choose traditional-style poles that reach shoulder-height, Lowe says.

Gaiters. If you are going to ski in snow that is higher than your ankles, Lowe suggests wearing gaiters, waterproof sheaths snapped on over your boots and pants legs. They'll keep the snow from getting in the tops of your boots.

Under- and outerwear. Dressing in layers allows you to adapt to changes in body temperature and weather conditions while you are skiing. Lowe says that she wears four layers for ski outings on cold, snowy days. Her first layer consists of tights and a long-sleeved undershirt, both made from moisture-wicking material (such as Capilene or Thermax). Then she adds a shirt, a wool sweater, and a jacket or fleece pullover on top. On the coldest days, she also wears insulated ski pants rather than basic ski pants. The jacket-and-pants outer layer, she says, should be made of material that is labeled waterproof or moisture resistant and breathable, such as Gore-Tex.

A hat. A warm hat is a must. Without one, you lose 25 to 40 percent of your body heat through your head. For cross-country skiing, you can wear the same kind of cap you'd wear for other outdoor winter sports—knit, fleece, and so forth.

A backpack. A backpack comes in handy for carrying any clothes that you shed as you warm up. Stock it with plenty of water and high-energy snacks. Snack on fruits, nuts, and sports bars, suggests Dr. Proctor. "Don't worry about the calories. You'll burn them off fast."

Sunscreen and sunglasses. Due in part to snow glare, the sun's rays are no less harmful in winter than in summer. Protect yourself by slathering exposed skin with sunscreen that has an SPF of 15 or higher. Also, wear sunglasses or goggles that screen out 100 percent of the sun's ultraviolet rays (the label should say so). Even on sunless days, eyewear safeguards your eyes against wind and snow, says Dr. Proctor.

FAT BLASTER

Skating is a technique in which you push your skis out to the sides rather than sliding them forward. The foot movements resemble ice skating. This type of cross-country skiing gives you an outstanding aerobic workout. But it is best done on snow where ski tracks haven't been set yet or on ground courses.

Cross-Country Skiing Workouts

Beginner	Intermediate	Experienced
25 to 45 minutes on a level or gently rolling trail, using the classic skiing technique	45 to 75 minutes on a prepared trail with rolling hills, using the classic technique or the skating technique	65 to 100 minutes on a packed, hilly trail, using the classic or skating technique; alternate 3 to 5 minutes of high-speed skiing (the fastest pace you can sustain) with 10 to 15 minutes of recovery skiing (in which your heart rate slows to about 65 percent of maximum)

CROSS-COUNTRY SKI MAC.

Calories Burned
254 to 339 per half-hour, depending on the intensity

Body-Shaping Potential
Tones the quadriceps, hamstrings, hips, buttocks, back, arms, shoulders, hips, and thighs

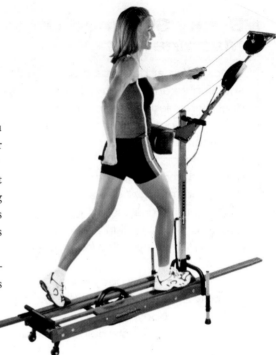

Here's what experts say you can expect if you use a cross-country ski machine as part of your body-shaping program.

▶ You'll get an all-around workout that works both your upper and lower body, raising your heart rate more and burning more calories than if you used exercise equipment that works just one or the other.

▶ You will work all your main muscles—quadriceps, hamstrings, hips, and glutes—as well as your back, arms, and shoulders.

On Your Feet

Unlike outdoor skiing, you needn't concern yourself with boots and bindings. Your feet will be inside toe cups on the machine, so you need only wear a pair of comfortable cross-trainers or running shoes. Jodi Paul, racquetball program director at the Allentown Racquetball and Fitness Club in Pennsylvania, prefers running shoes, because their pointier toes fit more snugly in the footholds.

Other Stuff You'll Need

If you're buying a cross-country ski machine for your home, you need to have a roomy area in which to use it. On most models, the skis extend beyond the simulator—figure on an overall length of about 8 feet and a width of about 3 feet.

Other machines are shuffle-type skiers that don't extend beyond the machine's body. But some users say they don't really simulate cross-country skiing, says Paul. "Still, they give a good workout and may be worth a look if space is a consideration."

Since fewer and fewer manufacturers are selling cross-country ski machines, most likely, you'll be using a machine at a gym or fitness center. Either way, here's what to look for when choosing one.

Real Women
SHOW YOU HOW

Becky Skimmed Off Pounds on a Ski Machine

Becky Warner bought a cross-country ski machine for her home because she wanted an alternative to her exercise video workouts. Then her marriage unraveled, and she hit the ski simulator with a renewed zeal.

"I'd take out all my frustrations on that poor machine," says Becky, age 46, a homemaker. A year later, Becky, who is 5 feet 5 inches tall, had gone from 154 to 127 pounds, dropping three dress sizes—from a 12 to a 6. Her hips are trimmer, plus her arms, back, and calves are shapelier. "I feel like I have more energy," she adds.

The marital crisis is over, but Becky continues using her ski simulator because it just wouldn't feel right if she didn't. "I'd feel guilty if I wasn't doing it," she says. "It's so much a part of my routine that if I don't do it, I miss it."

In addition to the body-shaping benefits, Becky says she also feels better mentally after a session on her ski machine. "I know I've done something good for my body," she says. "I feel like I've accomplished something. And it's cheaper than a shopping spree at the mall."

Consider the design. Ski machines come in two basic types. One, called a dependent system, links the skis with poles that you move back and forth or up and down with your hands. One foot moves forward, and the other automatically moves back. These machines are easy and safe to use, but they aren't as challenging as independent systems and may become boring.

An independent system works each foot separately and uses a cable, rather than poles, that you pull with your hands. This type of machine takes longer to learn, but the independent foot action is smoother and more enjoyable to use. Also, an independent machine forces you to use your upper body, so it gives you a more balanced workout.

Check the machine's features. Your ski simulator should be sturdy and have separate resistance settings for the legs and arms, so that you can increase the tension on either one or both as you become more proficient in the use of the machine. It also should have a mechanism to adjust for arm length. This will enable you to use the machine comfortably regardless of your height. Some machines have electronic monitors that tell you how fast you're moving, how many calories you're burning, how long you've been on the machine, and how far you've traveled.

Get more, pay more. If you find a store that sells cross-country ski simulators, be aware that they go for about $450 or more. Don't buy the bargain-basement machines.

Getting Started

Ski simulators are hard to get the hang of, but enthusiasts say they are worth the effort. Establishing a rhythm while moving your arms and legs is difficult.

"There's a big learning curve," says Laurie L. Tis, Ph.D., associate professor in the department of kinesiology and health at Georgia State University in Atlanta. "It takes practice."

Create tension. When you begin on the ski machine, make sure that there is some leg tension, even if it's only on the lowest setting. Otherwise, your feet may slide back too easily.

Warm up your legs. Warm up for 5 to 10 minutes before a workout on a ski simulator, recommends Dr. Tis. Start out at a leisurely walking pace for a few minutes, then gradually increase the speed or resistance for a few minutes and let this serve as your warmup. This will help you avoid strain and injury.

Give it time. Don't be discouraged if the machine initially feels as strange as dancing on a water bed. For most people, their first time on is not the time to judge whether they are going to like it or not. If you're considering buying a machine, try one out at your local Y or fitness center several times before making a purchase.

FAT BLASTER

The hardest thing to learn on this machine is how to develop a rhythm in which your arms and legs are moving in conjunction, not at odds with each other. Try perfecting just your leg movements at first, resting your hands on the handlebars or bumper pad in front of you until you do. Then gradually begin coordinating arm motion with that of your legs.

Cross-Country Ski Machine Workouts

Beginner
For the first 1 to 3 months, do only the lower-body movement of the machine. Aim for 30 strides per minute for 15 to 20 minutes, three times a week.

Intermediate
Add movement of your arms as well as your legs. Increase your pace by about 10 percent to 33 to 35 strides per minute. For the first month at this new rate, stick to the 15 to 20 minutes, three times a week, then gradually increase your time.

Experienced
Increase the resistance a couple of notches for your arm and leg movements. Aim for 40 strides a minute for 30 minutes, five times a week.

DANCING

Calories Burned

Per half-hour: ballroom, 105; modern, 147; country line, 150; aerobic, 201 to 276

Body-Shaping Potential

Tones the muscles of the calves, thighs, abdomen, buttocks, shoulders, arms, and upper back

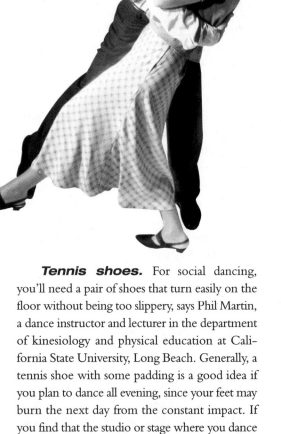

If you dance regularly, you can expect to see these results.

▶ Your entire lower body will be toned, especially your calves, thighs, buttocks, abdomen, and hips.

▶ You will strengthen the major muscles of your lower body, including your hamstrings, quadriceps, and gluteals. Some dance moves, such as pulling your partner forward in swing dancing, work the triceps, biceps, deltoids, and pectoral muscles.

▶ You'll lose weight and improve your cardiovascular fitness. Country line, folk, jazz, swing, samba, salsa, polka, and tap dancing may provide an aerobic workout. Other forms of dance, such as modern dancing or ballet, may be aerobic or not, depending on the moves and tempo.

On Your Feet

Okay, so it's time to put on your dancing shoes, which range from cross-trainer tennis shoes to ballet slippers to tap shoes, depending on the type of dance you do. When purchasing dance shoes (excluding tennis shoes), go to a specialty store where you can be fitted by an expert. Modern dance is often done barefoot. Here are some things to look for when you choose.

Tennis shoes. For social dancing, you'll need a pair of shoes that turn easily on the floor without being too slippery, says Phil Martin, a dance instructor and lecturer in the department of kinesiology and physical education at California State University, Long Beach. Generally, a tennis shoe with some padding is a good idea if you plan to dance all evening, since your feet may burn the next day from the constant impact. If you find that the studio or stage where you dance is sticky, you may need a leather or suede-soled shoe. Ballroom dance shoes are available, but they range from $70 to $150—a purchase you may want to put on hold until you've danced enough to know if it's right for you. Ballroom shoes are ideal for dancing, because they have suede soles

Real Women
SHOW YOU HOW

Lisa Dances Away the Night—And the Pounds

Lisa Deslauriers wasn't looking for a way to lose weight or get in shape. Recently divorced and feeling introverted, she wasn't even particularly interested in dating.

All that and a lot more began to change one afternoon when a coworker confided that he'd lost his dance partner, who had recently gotten engaged. "Do you want to try it?" he asked.

It took a few months of classes for Lisa to learn the Lindy Hop, a variation of swing dancing. Then, to the rhythm of the big band sounds of the 1930s and 1940s, Lisa found a new life.

"I basically started going out every single night. There were a lot of supportive people in the community willing to dance with a beginner, and it was fun. All of a sudden, I said, 'Wait a minute, I'm good at this!'" she recalls.

Over the next few years, the 33-year-old technical support whiz for a computer company found herself buying a new wardrobe for swing dancing. While she was purchasing new clothes for swing dancing, she realized that she also had to buy new clothes for work because she'd dropped a size or two from dancing.

"I had always worn clothes that were probably too big for me. But my body image changed, and I started wearing things that fit me more appropriately," she says.

Lisa was stunned to realize that she had lost 20 pounds despite an occasional ice cream cone after a night of spinning on the dance floor. But the weight-loss goals she realized were always secondary to the pure entertainment of swing.

"It became important to me to be able to dance the whole night and still be able to breathe easily enough to talk," she said.

that allow you to glide and turn but aren't too slippery. The rest of the shoe is usually made out of leather, which is lightweight and flexible. Keep the shoes clean with a shoe polish brush. Wax buildup on the soles of ballroom shoes can cause them to harden and lose friction.

Cowboy boots. For country line dancing, Martin says you can wear tennis shoes like the ones mentioned above or cowboy boots. "Look for cowboy boots with low heels, so you can dance more easily and comfortably," he suggests. Also, buying boots with leather material will keep your feet cool.

Socks. Socks should keep your shoes on without your feet slipping but definitely shouldn't make your shoes too snug, since your feet may swell a bit over the course of a night out on the dance floor. "Sometimes, a really thick sock can throw you off balance because it's too mushy," Martin warns. Socks that have cotton blend material help reduce slipping because they reduce sweat.

Ballet shoes. These run $20 to $30 and should be somewhat snugger than street shoes since they are leather and will stretch, says Lori Binkly, owner of Karabel Dancewear in Burbank, California. Your toe should touch the end when you're standing flat, but it should not be scrunched to fit in the shoe. If the shoes are too roomy, the leather will crinkle when you stand on your toes, she notes. Make sure the store has shoes that accommodate the width, not just the length, of your foot.

Tap shoes. Jazz tap shoes are available in an oxford and Mary Jane style, among others. Mary Janes are low-heeled strap shoes. Both the oxford and Mary Jane styles are best for beginners, since it is harder to learn in a high-heeled shoe, Binkly says. For $60 to $70, you can get such a shoe with the taps and rubber already in place, rather than having to take them to a shoemaker for customizing.

Other Stuff You'll Need

Modern and ballet dancers generally wear comfortable leotards, tights, and perhaps leg warmers. Square dancers and folk dancers may wear costumes, while country line dancers wear jeans and Western shirts. Aerobic and jazzercise dancers wear fitness clothing, from exercise bras to leggings or shorts.

Social dancing is generally done in casual street clothing, not exercise wear. Women shouldn't wear clothing made of a slippery fabric that may slide out of their partners' grasp or belts that could catch on an outstretched hand, cautions Martin.

Since dance is so varied, it's a good idea to call before the first class to be sure your footwear is permitted on the dance floor and your apparel is appropriate for the crowd.

To find beginning dance classes in your neighborhood, check your local newspaper, telephone book, or city parks and recreation activities bulletin.

Dancing Workouts

Beginner
Try a class that offers a slow waltz, fox-trot, or rumba. Dance at a level that allows easy conversation.

Intermediate
Dance the Viennese waltz, samba, or salsa.

Experienced
Do the polka or the East Coast swing, also called the jitterbug. You can also do country line dancing.

ELLIPTICAL TRAINING

Calories Burned

500 to 600 per hour

Body-Shaping Potential

Tones muscles of the entire lower body and burns fat

Here's what you can expect when you use an elliptical trainer regularly.

▶ When you move forward on the machine, you'll work your quadriceps and gluteus muscles.

▶ You'll tone and slim your entire lower body.

▶ You'll notice that your legs are shapelier than ever, since elliptical training uses all the muscles of the legs, large and small.

▶ You'll burn approximately 10 calories per minute while you work, and as a bonus, you'll continue to burn calories at a higher rate for a few hours afterward.

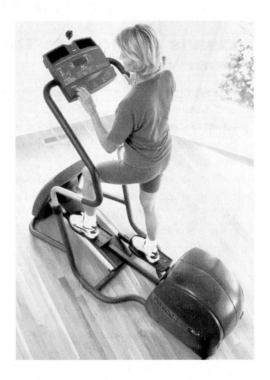

On Your Feet

Because your feet don't leave the elliptical trainer's surface, any lightweight athletic shoe will suffice, says Gregory Florez, owner of Fitness First, a personal training company in Chicago and Salt Lake City. Just be sure not to tie the laces too tightly, or your feet will start to feel numb.

To keep your feet dry and blister-free, pair those shoes up with athletic-wear socks of synthetic or cotton/synthetic fiber blends that breathe, advises Florez.

Other Stuff You'll Need

An elliptical trainer has various settings: resistance, speed, and, usually, ramp. You can program just one setting at a time or all three together.

As with a stationary bike, resistance on an elliptical trainer determines how much effort it will take for you to keep your feet moving. Ramp levels describe how high or low you've set the angle of the ellipse. For instance, a high ramp mimics hiking, while a low ramp mimics cross-country skiing. As you move, you determine the speed at which you move on the trainer. The resistance will, of course, affect the speed at which you *can* move, but how you respond to the resistance is under your control. You could, for example, choose a low resistance and move quickly, or you could put the resistance up high and not be able to move smoothly. Ideally, says Florez, you want to be

Real Women
SHOW YOU HOW

Lisa Is 45 Pounds Thinner—With a New Rear View

At the age of 35, Lisa Andruscavage found herself weighing 221 pounds and wearing a size 24. "At 5 feet 4 inches, my weight was really starting to affect my health," says Lisa, a mother of two. "In fact, I took 3 weeks off from work because I felt like my heart was actually tired, as if my body were going to shut down."

She hadn't tried exercise for years. "I'd had a number of miscarriages, and I'd stopped exercising when I was pregnant with my second child because I didn't want to overdo it," she says.

Lisa's first stop back at the gym was the stationary bicycles, but she didn't like them. "Boring," she thought.

Right next to the bicycles, however, was a piece of equipment Lisa had never seen before—an elliptical trainer. "I asked someone to show me how to use it," Lisa says. "I was able to do only 5 minutes, at level one with zero resistance. I thought, 'I'll never be able to do this.'"

Fortunately, Lisa stuck with it. "For me, the elliptical trainer is more interesting to use than the bike," Lisa says. "It didn't hurt my butt or my knees. Also, I have carpal tunnel syndrome, and the elliptical machine is easier on my hands than the other machines."

Within 4 months, Lisa was able to train for 30 to 35 minutes at a time, four times a week. "I keep the resistance low, but I move really quickly on a high ramp level," Lisa says. "That really works for me." The machine indicates that Lisa burns more than 300 calories per workout.

The results? In 1 year, Lisa has lost 45 pounds, and her percentage of body fat has gone down 14 percent. She's also down to a dress size of 16. "I've lost most of the extra weight in my legs and butt," she says. "In fact, many people notice my weight loss from behind. They'll come up and say, 'I was behind you, and I didn't recognize you.'"

able to move at a comfortable, moderate speed, interspersed with occasional bursts of high intensity as well as high speeds.

Quality elliptical trainers are expensive and may cost up to six times as much as a treadmill or stationary bike, putting them out of range for many home exercisers. So most likely, you'll use a trainer at a gym or fitness center, at least at first. If you fall in love with elliptical training and want to buy a machine for your home, here are some buying tips from experts.

Go for range. Look for a variety of ramp settings and intensity levels in an elliptical machine. If the ellipse itself isn't expansive and doesn't offer ramp and intensity changes, then the workout isn't nearly as effective.

The Precor EFX models, for example, use an oval-shaped collection of gears, pedals, and flywheels that allows the legs to move in their full range of motion, giving you a good workout. At retail, they sell for approximately $2,000 to $2,700. If you try less expensive machines, with less of an elliptical shape, you may find that you don't get the same range of motion, says Florez.

If you can afford it, consider a model with a control panel that offers various preprogrammed courses and records how many calories you've burned.

Skip the handles. Some machines come with handles that allow you to move your arms back and forth—with resistance—while you're on the elliptical machine. "That doesn't increase calorie burning very much," says Florez. "To burn more calories, it's much more effective to buy a machine without handles and work your legs at a higher intensity without leaning on your arms."

Try various settings. As with a treadmill or stationary bike, you'll want to get a sense of how the machine feels at different settings. Try different combinations of ramp and speed settings. Also, vary the resistance, which enables you to work at different levels of intensity. The higher the resistance, the more power you'll need to exert to get your feet moving.

Measure twice, buy once. Elliptical trainers are long—up to 5 feet long and over 4 feet tall at their highest point. Measure the machine you're going to buy and the space in which you plan to use it.

Don comfortable clothes. Elliptical trainers don't require a special outfit. As with most workouts, your best bet is a layer or two of loose-fitting, comfortable clothing made of fabrics that wick sweat away. That way, you can peel off a layer as you work up a sweat. After a few workouts, you'll find what works best for you, says Florez.

FAT BLASTER

If you want to stay in shape for weekend hiking excursions, or if you just want to reap the benefits that hiking brings to your quadriceps and butt, keep the elliptical trainer's ramp setting on high and increase the intensity on the machine, which will simulate climbing.

Elliptical Training Workouts

Beginner	Intermediate	Experienced
Two or three times a week for 10 to 20 minutes at a time in a slow rhythm	Two or three times a week for at least 20 minutes, using a pre-programmed workout that doesn't include intervals	Two or three times a week for 20 to 60 minutes of interval training, either pre-programmed or self-directed

GARDENING

Calories Burned

Per 10 minutes: planting seedlings, 48; hoeing, 62; digging, 86

Body-Shaping Potential

This head-to-toe workout tones arms, shoulders, chest, back, buttocks, abdomen, and legs.

Gardening provides excellent whole-body exercise, says Richard Cotton, chief exercise physiologist for the American Council on Exercise in San Diego. Here's how.

▶ Walking and other large-muscle movements provide an aerobic workout. Gardening activities like raking, sweeping, hoeing, and shoveling are the most aerobic because they are sustained activities.

▶ You'll exercise your back, chest, abdomen, buttocks, legs, arms, and shoulders with the pushing and pulling movements of digging and tilling. Your arms and shoulders will get exercise as you plant, weed, and do sit-down digging. Finally, you'll exercise your legs and buttocks with the repetitive up-and-down of moving along a flower or vegetable bed.

▶ Gardening offers the kind of sustained, moderate, fat-burning workout that, when performed three to five times a week, can help you lose weight and keep it off.

which can be very comfortable for certain foot types.

On Your Feet

Because of the many positions your feet will be in as you garden, you'll want to find shoes that have flexible toes and rear-foot support. Also keep in mind that you'll want shoes that will protect you from bug bites. You might want to check out a pair of gardening clogs,

Other Stuff You'll Need

The gardening tools and supplies you need will depend on the size and character of your garden.

Tools. One day you may very well need an industrial-strength soil tiller to dig up the acre behind your house, but for starters, stick to a few

Real Women
SHOW YOU HOW

Gardening Keeps Kate Slim and Young

Kate Flynn lost 25 pounds, wears a size 6 or 8, and looks more like 39 than 49—thanks to gardening, her favorite form of "exercise."

"During my childhood and young adult years, I'd always been self-conscious about my weight," says Kate, who is a clinical therapist and single mom. "All my female relatives were chubby, and I saw myself gaining weight and starting to look just like them."

Kate tried running, aerobics, and even walking, but without much success. "I found I couldn't run every day," she says. "And it was hard on my knees—I felt like I was killing my body. I enjoyed aerobics classes, but raising two young sons on my own made it hard to get to class. And raising two growing boys, I couldn't afford it."

When Kate bought a little ranch home for herself and her boys, she plunged into gardening in a big way—with big results.

"I was determined to make the most of the space—I ripped out parts of the lawn and planted beds of medicinal herbs, shrubs, and ornamental grasses, plus a few vegetables. There are three of us, but you know how kids feel about vegetables and gardening," she adds.

Make no mistake about it, says Kate: Gardening is a real workout. "I'm moving constantly—pulling weeds, carrying buckets of mulch and clippings, raking the soil flat."

Kate says working out has really helped keep her firm. "My legs were always heavy, but now they're much slimmer."

Plus, she looks much younger than other women her age. "When I go out, people who meet me for the first time always think I'm 37, 38, or 39. They never think I'm the age I am."

hand tools such as a shovel, cultivator, and hoe, says Cotton. As your ambitions and competence grow, work up to long-handled, stand-up tools, which give you more of a full-body workout.

Other equipment. Find yourself a cushiony mat to kneel or sit on while weeding, gardening gloves to protect against abrasions and keep dirt at bay, and clothing that breathes when you sweat in the heat and that keeps you cozy in cooler weather. Don't forget to wear at least some sunscreen and a hat to ward off damaging ultraviolet rays. Kathi Colen, urban agriculture coordinator for SLUG, the San Francisco League of Urban Gardeners, goes even further. She never gardens without sunglasses, a wide-brimmed hat, long sleeves, and long pants, for allover protection from both sun exposure and wayward twigs and branches.

Getting Started

Whether you have a container garden on your porch or a large plot of land to work with, here's how to get started.

Set reasonable goals. Don't expect to dig and plant your garden all at once, says Suzanne DeJohn, horticulture staff coordinator at the National Gardening Association in Burlington, Vermont. "Do one thing at a time, a little at a time."

Choose the right time. During hot weather, avoid working in stressful midday heat by gardening before 10:00 A.M. and after 2:00 P.M. Also, try working when you're usually most energetic. If you're a morning person, hit the dirt when the sun comes up. If you don't get revved up until later in the day, save gardening for the late afternoon or evening.

Drink plenty of water. To avoid dehydration, which can lead to fatigue and muscle cramps, have a glass of water before you begin gardening, and sip frequently from a jug or water bottle while you're out there, advises Barbara Ainsworth, Ph.D., associate professor of exercise science and director of the Prevention Research Center at the University of South Carolina in Columbia.

Aim for variety. Engaging in a variety of movements every time you garden trains a variety of muscles, making you stronger and more toned overall, says Cotton. It also reduces the risk of overstressing specific muscles and joints. For example, dig for 10 minutes, then switch to planting or weeding, then to watering, and then to tossing weeds and twigs into a basket.

Bend and lift smartly. Gardening can put a real strain on your lower back, says Dr. Ainsworth. Instead of bending at the waist to weed or plant, squatting down on one knee with the other knee bent is a safer, healthier posture. When lifting, use your legs instead of your back.

Hold tools up close. Even the lightest tools can strain your muscles when they're used for the repetitive motions of gardening. To reduce the strain, hold tools closer to your body, suggests Dr. Ainsworth. Rather than stretching for weeds and placing your back in an unsupported position, dig up the ones that are nearby with a hand shovel held close to your side. Then either switch sides after you've pulled all the weeds that are close to you or do one side of a row and then come back down the other side. To include more stretching while gardening, reach with your whole torso, making sure your back is supported under your feet and legs, she adds.

Gardening Workouts

Beginner	Intermediate	Experienced
Weeding or planting seeds or seedlings for 10 minutes at a time	Tilling with a long-handled tiller or hoeing or other chores for 30 minutes at a time	Digging or spreading fertilizer or mulch or other chores for 45 minutes at a time, 5 days a week

HIKING

Calories Burned

250 per half-hour

Body-Shaping Potential

Tones the legs and buttocks; will also increase aerobic endurance

Physiologically, hiking is walking turned up a notch or two. Here's how you can benefit.

▶ You'll burn more calories by hiking than by walking, since climbing hills or walking on uneven terrain takes more energy.

▶ When you carry a pack of some kind (which most people do), the extra pounds further pump up your calorie burning.

▶ You'll give your quadriceps, hamstrings, gluteus maximus, and gluteus minimus a good workout, since hill walking forces your leg and thigh muscles to work even harder and more intensely than walking on flat terrain.

▶ If you use hiking poles, you'll tone your arm and back muscles, too.

On Your Feet

You don't have to hoist a heavy overnight pack and sleep in a tent to hike. But you do need more than ordinary sneakers. You can get by with running or walking shoes, especially for short hikes on relatively flat terrain. But your feet will be a lot happier in hiking boots, especially if you have problems with weak ankles or balance.

Look for boots or trail shoes with lugged rubber soles. "You need a shoe with traction over rocks, dirt, leaves, and tree roots—all of which are slippery, especially when wet," says Dan Heil, Ph.D., assistant professor of exercise physiology at Montana State University in

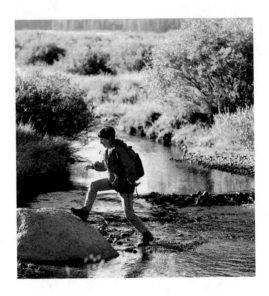

Bozeman. "And you need ankle support for stability." Whatever you do, don't wear loafers.

Other Stuff You'll Need

Like fitness walking, hiking calls for a few other essentials.

Proper clothing. Thinking blue jeans? Think again. "Jeans are 100 percent cotton, which holds moisture against the skin if it gets wet from inside or outside the body," says Dr. Heil. "Instead, wear nylon shorts or hiking pants and pullovers made from fabrics such as polypropylene or CoolMax, which keep moisture away from your body and dry quickly. In extremely cold weather, wear three layers. Use fabrics such as CoolMax, polypropylene, or ThermaStat blends as an inner layer to wick moisture away from the skin. As a middle layer, insulate by trapping a layer of warm air next to your body with fleece, wool, or BiPolar fleece. The outer layer should shield you from weather extremes. Wind jackets and pants of either Gore-Tex or Gore-Tex and fleece are all good outer protectors." If the weather is clear and only mildly cold, an inner and middle layer will suffice, adds Dr. Heil. You can find these clothes in sporting goods stores.

"If it's cool enough to wear a jacket, then you also need gloves and a hat, since the largest source of heat loss is through the head and extremities," says Dr. Heil.

An extra pair of socks. If you're going on a long hike—more than half a day or so—wear two pairs of socks. The first (closest to your feet) should be made of a lightweight material that wicks away moisture, such as CoolMax. The outer layer should be made of a thicker material that protects your feet from rubbing against your shoe, like wool. "Switch to a new pair of both layers of socks about midway through the trip," says Dr. Heil. "It really feels better and is good for your skin."

Food. Okay, if you're just going for a 15-minute loop through the park, you will probably survive without something to eat. But if you're heading out for a couple of hours or longer, count on getting hungry. "You want snacks that are high in complex carbohydrates, such as granola bars, bananas, or a sandwich," says Dr. Heil.

Water. Anytime you exercise for an hour or more, you need to drink water to avoid even mild dehydration. So always carry bottled water or a water purifier. "Never drink water from a stream or creek, because you don't know what might be upstream," says Dr. Heil. "Waste from livestock or wildlife may be just a few hundred yards away, or decomposing animals could be nearby, and you don't want to drink water that's passing over those areas before it makes its way down to you."

A walking stick. You can buy one, or you can simply use a sturdy stick you find on your trail (unless you're hiking in the desert). "Walking sticks are great if you have a back problem, bad knees, or trouble with balance," says Dr. Heil. "It's a third point on the ground. In fact, experienced hikers prefer two poles, which turn them into four-legged creatures." And they come in handy when crossing small streams.

One avid pole-user is Diane Benedict, manager and trip leader for Mountain Fit, an organization in Bozeman that plans hiking adventures. "When descending, I find poles helpful to lessen the impact on my knees," she says. "And using one or two poles turns hiking into a great upper- and lower-body workout."

A map. Unless you can actually see the entire area that you're walking *while* you're walking, you need a map. "Call hiking clubs, walking clubs, a visitors bureau, or a park headquarters where you plan to hike," suggests Dr. Heil.

Hiking Workouts

Beginner	Intermediate	Experienced
20 to 30 minutes of hiking on a trail or a beach three times a week	40 minutes of hiking 5 or 6 days a week, plus a long hike (60 minutes) up and over a mountain on Saturday	Longer hikes on rockier terrain, which take 2 to 4 hours; for highly experienced hikers, adventures that last for more than 4 hours

HOUSEWORK

Calories Burned
30 to 50 per 10-minute period

Body-Shaping Potential
Tones arms, shoulders, chest, back, buttocks, abdomen, and legs

Because it engages all of your major muscle groups, housework builds strength, endurance, and flexibility, says Thomas P. Martin, Ph.D., professor in the health, fitness, and sport department at Wittenberg University in Springfield, Ohio. Here's how.

▶ Picking up clutter and carrying it from one room to another and—an even greater challenge—carrying it up and down flights of stairs works the muscles of your arms, shoulders, legs, and buttocks, Dr. Martin explains, while your back and abdominal muscles stabilize your body.

▶ You'll primarily work your upper body by pushing a vacuum, but walking with your vacuum from one end of your home to the other works your legs and midsection.

▶ Scrubbing a floor or washing windows helps maintain strength in your arms and back, while the stretching motion maintains flexibility, says Russell Pate, Ph.D., an exercise physiologist at the University of South Carolina in Columbia.

Getting Started

Anyone who has spent a weekend spring-cleaning only to wake up stiff and sore on Monday morning knows that even informal types of exercise call for certain precautions. Here's what you need to know.

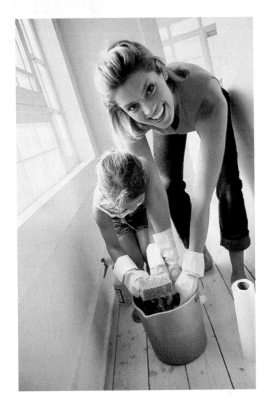

Take it slow. Work yourself up slowly to doing housework for extensive periods, especially strenuous tasks. "Don't be a spring-cleaning athlete," Dr. Martin advises. "People make this mistake all the time. They give their whole house a big cleaning once a year, but if they haven't done so since last spring, they're going to end up aching all over."

Alternate activities. To avoid overworking particular muscles, switch from one task to another, suggests Dr. Pate. "It's a good idea to move the work around to various muscle groups and move the stress around from joint to joint and tissue to tissue." For example,

Real Women SHOW YOU HOW

She Dismissed Her Housekeeper— And Shaped Up

While in her late forties, Julie Cooney became determined to start exercising regularly. She had put on extra pounds during menopause, and while she didn't feel terribly overweight, she did feel awfully out of shape.

So when Julie's cleaning lady announced her retirement, Julie decided not to replace her. Instead, she reclaimed her mop, vacuum, and dirty laundry, and she turned cleaning her house into an exercise regimen.

"I try to do everything very deliberately," says Julie, now 61. "I have three floors to vacuum, plus hardwood floors everywhere to mop. I'm constantly picking things up and climbing up and down stairs to put them away. When I'm doing laundry, I throw everything on the floor. Then I sort it all out with a kind of ballet movement, bending down for each piece and throwing it in a sweeping motion, whites to the right and darks to the left.

"There's always housework to be done, so I figure I may as well get the most out of it," Julie says. "It really is a wonderful way to stay in shape. I feel great, better than I felt in my forties."

do a little bit of vacuuming, then put in a load of laundry, and then scrub the bathroom sink.

Position yourself properly. The bending, lifting, twisting, reaching, and other often demanding movements of housework can play havoc with muscles and joints, says Dr. Pate. "My general advice would be not to force yourself into positions you're not accustomed to or that feel abnormal. In particular, don't do so over and over again or over a long period of time."

Bend and lift smartly. Housework can put a real strain on your vulnerable lower back. Use proper technique to protect yourself: Bend and lift with your legs, not your back.

Housework Workouts

Low Intensity	Moderate Intensity	High Intensity
Doing laundry, making beds, ironing, washing dishes, putting away groceries, cooking, vacuuming	Sweeping the garage, sidewalk, or outside of the house; washing windows; mopping vigorously	Moving household furniture, carrying heavy boxes, climbing or carrying items up stairs

INLINE SKATING

Calories Burned
340 to 476 an hour, depending on how vigorous the skating

Body-Shaping Potential
Tones the legs, especially the calves and inner and outer thighs, and the buttocks and abdomen

If you're game, here's what you can expect from regular inline skating.

▶ You'll tone and strengthen your lower body and torso, including your calves, thighs, buttocks, and to a lesser degree, your tummy.

▶ You'll get a cardiovascular workout roughly comparable to running, without stressing your joints as much.

▶ You'll burn about as much fat and calories as treadmill running, stepping, or rowing but will have a lot more fun along the way.

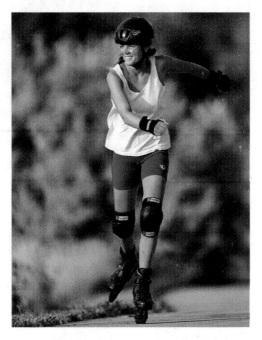

On Your Feet

Inline skates are nothing like the metal contraptions you clamped to your play shoes with a skate key when you were in grade school. Basically, an inline skate is more like a sturdy ice skate with a series of wheels, bearings, and a brake built into a double-shelled boot with a buckle and lacing.

The number one criterion in choosing a skate is comfort, says Kalinda Mathis, executive director of the International Inline Skating Association in Wilmington, North Carolina. Since skate prices start at about $100 and a quality pair of skates will cost between $150 and $300, it makes sense to rent several styles and brands before you commit. Some local sports equipment shops will rent them by the day.

Be sure to get women's skates for women's feet. Most women prefer skates designed for women's feet, notes Mathis. They're built on a narrower last (the mold used for making footwear) than men's skates.

Start with a recreational skate. Compared to recreational skates, fitness skates are lighter, have a lower-cut boot, and larger wheels (76 to 80 versus 72 to 76 millimeters). As a beginner, you'll probably want to start on a recreational skate; later, you may want to switch to a more high-performance fitness skate should you commit to power workouts on wide, smooth surfaces.

Other Stuff You'll Need

When you walk or run, you're generally traveling at a speed of 3 to 8 miles per hour—a

Real Women
SHOW YOU HOW

Nicole Skated Off Her "Stress Weight"

Nicole G. Lambros, 34, knew it before her doctor broke the news. At 5 feet 2 inches and 140 pounds, the makeup artist and hairdresser realized she was carrying too much "stress weight," put on after her divorce as she adjusted to a cross-country move and life as a single mom.

So one morning, Nicole put on her tennis shoes and started walking. Walking became jogging. Pretty soon, she was doing 2 miles a day, but she was bored. So she slipped into her son's inline skates.

"My son had a pair of Rollerblades, and when he went to his dad's for the summer, I put them on and off I went," she says with a giggle.

Nicole had an edge: She had figure-skated as a child, so inline skating came easily. In fact, she wowed a group of single, divorced men, who were stunned by how quickly she learned to balance, turn, and stop. "You've bladed before!" they accused her.

"I loved it from the very first minute," she admits. The only adjustment she had to make from figure skating was braking, which is done with the back of inline skates and from the front in figure skates.

Within 6 months, Nicole began to notice major changes in her body, especially in her buttocks, but also in her legs, abdominals, lower back, arms, and chest. She wasn't dieting, but her weight was dropping—10 pounds, 15, then 20 within the year.

"Clients of mine who are personal trainers were saying, 'What are you doing? You look great!'" says the beautician. Her doctor was amazed—and very pleased.

Nicole now skates every morning, and she loves the way she looks and feels. But she says the changes in her life have gone beyond the physical.

"Skating opened up my mind. It's my natural Prozac," she says.

---

pretty leisurely clip. Inline skaters travel on hard surfaces at much faster speeds—anywhere from 10 to 25 miles per hour. Pebbles, deep sidewalk cracks, or other objects can trip up your wheels. Sooner or later, you'll fall. Unless you wear protective gear, you can fracture your wrist, arm, or collarbone, cautions Richard A. Schieber, M.D.,

of the National Center for Injury Prevention and Control in Atlanta. Here's what you'll need.

Wrist guards. When you fall, you tend to fall forward, putting your hand out to break your fall. Padded, plastic wrist guards dissipate the impact—you slide along the ground on impact, saving your wrist from a sprain or fracture from the impact. "Wrist guards are absolutely necessary," says Dr. Schieber.

Knee and elbow pads. Injuries to the knees and elbows are less common than injuries to the wrists, but you still want to protect them from scrapes and other injuries. Protective pads help cushion your fall so you don't leave part of your skin behind.

Helmets. Since a collision with the pavement or a vehicle can be catastrophic, you want to protect your brain. A biking helmet might be better than an inline skating helmet, because it must meet certain standards. All bicycle helmets made or sold in the United States have to meet federal safety standards set by the Consumer Product Safety Commission (CPSC). Dr. Schieber recommends a CPSC-certified bicycle helmet, but he says any helmet is better than none.

Clothing. What you wear to skate should accommodate your pads (jeans may not be comfortable with knee pads) and otherwise be comfortable and nonrestrictive. Most skaters choose exercise shorts on warm days or leggings on chilly days, plus comfortable tops that allow them to freely pump their arms.

Getting Started

Inline skating may look easy, but don't let that fool you into thinking you can just strap on a pair of skates and hit the sidewalk. "Learning some basic moves and wearing the right equipment can greatly minimize your chances of hurting yourself," says Craig Young, M.D., medical director of sports medicine at the Medical College of Wisconsin in Milwaukee.

First, learn how to brake. Proper braking on inline skates isn't difficult, says Mathis, but it doesn't come as second nature to newcomers. Save yourself time—and potential bruises: Call a sporting goods store that sells inline skates or your local parks and recreation department, and sign up for an individual or group lesson, so an instructor can show you how to glide, stride, and most important, stop.

Find a smooth, safe place to get started. Carolyn Bradley, of Wayne, Pennsylvania, an examiner for the International Inline Skating Assocation instructor certification program, recommends an empty parking lot, maybe early on a weekend morning, or an uncrowded bike path. "Definitely don't start skating on the street," she says.

The ideal place for any inline skating is a roller rink, adds Dr. Schieber.

Relax. Bend your knees and keep your hands in front of you as you glide your feet slowly and smoothly in front of each other, says Mathis. The rhythm will soon come easily to you.

Inline Skating Workouts

Beginner	**Intermediate**	**Experienced**
Skate for 15 to 25 minutes, alternating between 10 slow strides and 10 fast strides.	Skate for 40 minutes, starting with 10 fast, then 10 slow strides. Then do 20 fast strides and 10 slow strides.	Skate for 60 minutes using shorter, faster strokes. Abbreviate the glide between strokes.

JOGGING AND TREADMILL RUNNING

Calories Burned

102 per mile

Body-Shaping Potential

Firms the calves, thighs, buttocks, and to a lesser extent, the abdomen

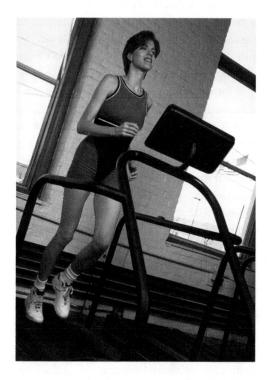

Whether you jog on a treadmill or through a dew-sprinkled park, slow running provides a wealth of physical payoffs.

▶ You work both the large and the small muscle groups of your calves, thighs, buttocks, and hips, and in a less pronounced way, your waist and abdominal muscles.

▶ You burn calories and use up fat stores, big time.

▶ You'll raise your metabolic rate even after your running shoes are back in the closet. According to researchers at the University of Colorado, the resting metabolic rates of middle-aged women runners stayed steady as they grew older, while sedentary women gained weight and body fat as their resting metabolisms slowed. In the long run, older runners burn up to 600 additional calories a week (equal to 9 pounds a year!) even when they're at rest. "That doesn't even count the calories burned when they run," notes Pamela P. Jones, research assistant professor of kinesiology and applied physiology at the University of Colorado at Boulder.

On Your Feet

Fortunately for joggers, manufacturers have come a long way in designing shoes to accommodate the sizes and running styles of virtually any woman, at prices that generally range from $50 to $100. Here's what to look for, according to Ellen Glickman-Weiss, Ph.D., associate professor of exercise physiology in the department of exercise, leisure, and sports at Kent State University in Kent, Ohio.

Shoes for your feet. Reading running-shoe reviews can help you decide which of the dozens of shoe makes and models might best meet your needs, says Dr. Glickman-Weiss. Also consult knowledgeable salesclerks at sporting goods stores or athletic shoe stores. Take your old shoes along. Worn spots show whether you run more on the outside or the inside of your foot and which areas need the most support.

Enough wiggle room. A wide toebox is vital to give the front of your foot enough room when the force of your foot is pushed forward. Women with wide feet may want to check out running shoes designed specifically for women, from companies like Rykä, New Balance, and Saucony.

All-weather, all-surface tread and materials. If you're going to be running in rain and snow, look for a shoe made from weather-tight fabric, with a hard-core outer tread. If you're a treadmill runner, this isn't important.

Replacements, as needed. Buy a new pair of shoes every 6 months or 600 miles.

At that point, the shoes start to fall apart, even if they still look good. You can prolong the life of your running shoes by wearing them only to run.

Run Smarter

You don't need to run every day. Running too fast—or too often—can increase the risk of injuries. Three to 5 days a week is fine. And if you're just starting out, you shouldn't run more than 15 miles a week. At that point, the stresses on your muscles, joints, tendons, and ligaments outweigh the body-shaping benefits. According to Dr. Glickman-Weiss, there are other, better

Real Women SHOW YOU HOW

A Second Attempt at Jogging Did the Trick

Cynthia Smith didn't set out to lose weight. "I really just wanted to do something to improve my overall health," says the 45-year-old sales executive.

Nevertheless, Cynthia knew she could stand to lose a few pounds. "I had some extra weight around my hips and abdomen, and I felt heavy," she recalls. So she began to search for an exercise routine that would fit into her busy traveling schedule and be enjoyable. "I did some running in my twenties and really loved it," says Cynthia. So she decided to try it again.

Cynthia's renewed efforts at jogging paid off, physically and mentally. "After only a few months of jogging, I started feeling trimmer and more toned," she remembers. "I went from 134 to 124 pounds, I dropped a dress size, and my clothes fit me better."

"Plus, my runs are therapeutic," adds Cynthia. "They clear my head, and I get ideas." She doesn't always feel like lacing up her running shoes and heading out. "But I always feel better physically and emotionally after I'm done," she says. "Jogging after a hard day at work is a tremendous tension reliever. Everything that builds up during the day just sort of vaporizes."

ways to maximize your efforts than going all-out, all the time. Here's how.

Increase your weekly distance by no more than 10 percent a week. If you're jogging 3 days a week for 30 minutes a day, for example, and covering 3 miles, increase by no more than 1 mile total the first week, and so forth.

Stick to flat, smooth surfaces. If you run outdoors, you can run longer while minimizing impact if you stick to a soft, smooth, unbanked cinder track or an artificial surface. The same goes for soft, smooth dirt trails. Avoid asphalt and concrete.

Alternate jogging with other activities. Swimming, water aerobics, cycling, stairclimbing, rowing, or cross-country skiing gives your feet and legs a welcome respite from the constant pounding of running, while working other muscle groups than running would alone.

Treadmill Tips

If you find that rain and snow keep you from jogging, try treadmill running at a gym. If you find yourself sticking to it (and can afford it), consider purchasing a treadmill for home. To save money, shop at a secondhand sports equipment store.

Choose a body-friendly model. Some treadmills have a built-in suspension, like shock absorbers on a car, to minimize the impact on weak hips or knees, says Edmund Burke, Ph.D., professor of exercise science at the University of Colorado in Colorado Springs.

These machines approximate the impact of running on a soft surface, says Dr. Glickman-Weiss. They're also sturdier and better able to accommodate heavier walkers and runners than lightweight units that you can stow under a bed.

Go for a "test jog." If you decide to buy, go to a reputable fitness showroom dressed for action. Run on many treadmills, looking for a shock-absorbing platform, a belt wide and long enough for you, and handrails you like.

Know you can stop. So you can stop without risking an injury, make sure the treadmill has a device that will immediately stop the belt in case you run into trouble, advises Dr. Burke.

FAT BLASTER

The next time you see a charity run announced in the newspaper, sign up. The competition, free T-shirt, and opportunity to help raise money for causes like breast cancer, arthritis, or Alzheimer's research will motivate you to stick with your program.

Jogging Workouts

Beginner	Intermediate	Experienced
Alternate jogging and walking for 20 minutes a day, 3 to 5 days a week.	Jog for 40 minutes, at least 4 or 5 days a week.	Jog for an hour, up to five times a week, not to exceed 30 miles a week. Beyond 30 miles, there is really no extra benefit, and your risk of injury increases.

JUMPING ROPE

Calories Burned

110 to 130 per 10-minute session

Shaping Potential

A high-level calorie burner. Firms up the buttock and thigh muscles. Also develops calf muscles.

Women who want to lose weight are ideal candidates for jumping rope, says Ken Solis, M.D., an emergency room physician at Beaver Dam Community Hospital in Greenfield, Wisconsin, and author of *Ropics*, a book of exercises he developed for the jump rope. Among the rewards:

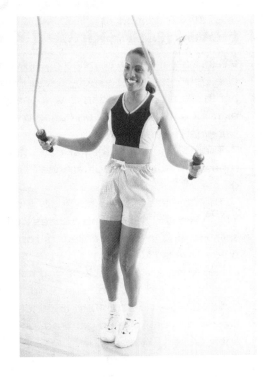

▶ You'll burn calories—lots of them. Jumping rope is on a par with running when it comes to calorie burn.

▶ You'll improve endurance, coordination, balance, and timing.

▶ You'll strengthen your bones as well as your muscles; this is a great bonus, because it helps prevent osteoporosis.

On Your Feet

Since you're going to be doing a lot of bouncing on the balls of your feet, wearing the right shoes is important. Otherwise, you could sprain an ankle or tear a tendon. You'll need a quality pair of aerobic or cross-training shoes to give you cushioning and support in all the right places, says exercise physiologist Carla Sottovia, assistant fitness director at the Cooper Fitness Center in Dallas. When you're in the store, cast your inhibitions to the wind and jump up and down to make sure the shoes fit right. As for those old tennis shoes, running shoes, or sneakers in your closet—use them for other sports, she says.

Other Stuff You'll Need

Once upon a time, an old clothesline may have served as a jump rope. Now you have many more choices—and it's also important to choose the right bra and mat. Here are some of the possibilities.

Spring for the swivel. The rope should swivel within the handles or at the handles, so that the rope doesn't twist on itself while you're jumping, says Dr. Solis.

Choose right. Jump ropes are made of many materials. Starting out, you might choose a segmented rope (otherwise known as a beaded rope) or a rope made of woven

Real Women
SHOW YOU HOW

How Heidi Skipped 4 Inches off Her Hips

Heidi Zarder was a certified group exercise instructor. Now, being an exercise instructor is not exactly a sedentary job. But even so, after Heidi had her third child, she began to wonder whether she would ever get rid of the extra pounds she'd put on during pregnancy. Her normal workout routine just wasn't getting results.

Then, 8 months after her daughter was born, she started jumping rope. "It made all the difference," says Heidi. "In 1 month, I lost 4 inches off my hips."

The new exercise was actually the result of Heidi's profession. "The local YMCA wanted me to lead classes that mixed different forms of exercise," says Heidi. "One week called for rope jumping. In order to teach, I had to practice myself."

Heidi had a wood deck behind her house, and that became her happy jumping ground. "I made sure I didn't jump or bounce too hard," says Heidi. "I would work on it for 10 to 15 minutes, watching myself in the reflection of the patio door. Then I'd get tired, go inside, and come back out to practice again when I felt ready."

Heidi knew she had reached a plateau in her efforts to lose weight, and skipping rope was the boost she needed to lose the last few pounds. "Many people who go to step and aerobics classes never lose any weight," notes Heidi. "That's because they reach a plateau and need something to kick in a higher amount of calorie burning. Rope skipping can blast you through the plateau."

One unforeseen problem, however, was bladder control. "After three kids, bouncing up and down could trigger leakage," says Heidi. "To handle this, I just avoided drinking anything with caffeine. I limited how much water I drank before I worked out. Instead, I drank plenty of water *while* I was exercising."

Now, when she teaches aerobics classes, Heidi includes rope skipping. It has been a popular addition to her classes at a local college. "It's great for coordination," says Heidi. "But most everyone uses it as a tool for weight loss. It simply burns a lot of calories."

cotton or synthetic material. The segmented or beaded ropes have a nylon cord at the center that is strung with cylindrical plastic beads that look like hollow noodles. A woven rope, made of nylon, cotton, or polypropylene, resembles the old-fashioned kind of jump rope, and it won't sting as much if you happen to swat your back, Dr. Solis notes from personal experience.

After you've advanced a bit, you might choose a speed rope or licorice rope. They're made from vinyl plastic, and they're light and fast. Leather ropes are just as fast as speed ropes, but they wear out sooner. Some advanced jump ropers who are in very good physical condition choose weighted ropes that can weigh up to 6 pounds. Needless to say, you don't want a weighted rope until you're very confident about your swinging and timing, says Dr. Solis.

Measure for leisure. When a rope is the right length, you can hold it at waist level and hardly move your hands, and it will clear your head and feet with no problem. (If you have to circle your arms around, the rope's too short; if it bounces and hits your ankles, it's too long.) To get a comfortable length, stand with one or two feet in the middle of the rope, then lift the handles as high as they'll go. If they reach your armpits, you have what you want, says Dr. Solis. Some ropes are adjustable, and others can be shortened just by putting in a couple of overhand knots near the handles.

Cradle your top. You probably know by now whether you're more comfortable in an exercise bra—but this is a sport where you might even want two. Women who take a bra size 36 or larger usually do best by layering two

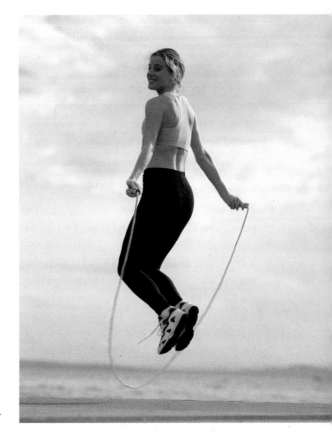

running bras on top of each other, and then wearing a close-fitting T-shirt or tank on top of that, says Sottovia.

Find the space. "Even though it's convenient to skip rope at home, it's sometimes hard to find enough room above you and around you," says Dr. Solis. If you're average height, you'll need at least a 9-foot ceiling, with plenty of space around you. The lawn won't work, because the rope gets tangled in the grass, and carpet slows you down. So you might head for the basement, garage, or patio. That's fine, as long as you're on a surface that has a little give to it, like wood or hard rubber, says Dr. Solis. You don't want to jump on hard concrete or tile, he warns. Those surfaces don't give you any bounce, and they're murder on your joints.

Go to the mat. You can convert a thick carpet into a jump-friendly surface by using a plastic mat that is usually sold to be placed underneath an office desk or chair, says Dr. Solis. These are available at larger office supply stores.

To convert the floor in a garage or spare room into a jump-friendly surface, invest in plastic interlocking tiles, says Budd Pickett, executive director of the United States Amateur Jump Rope Federation (USAJRF). These are not soft mats, but flooring used in indoor courts for sports such as volleyball, gymnastics, and jump roping, he explains. To locate a store near you that sells interlocking tiles, write to Sport Court at 939 South 700 West, Salt Lake City, UT 84104.

A hard rubber mat or flooring is good, too, according to Dr. Solis. Avoid squishy aerobics mats because they have too much give, he adds.

FAT BLASTER

There are many variations on jumping rope, and if you observe some advanced rope-skippers, you'll get some ideas on how to make your jump-rope workout even more interesting and challenging. One variation is the heel dig jump: With each jump, you bring one leg in front of your body as if you were digging in your heel. It looks like a variation on a Cossack dance without the deep squat or the funny hat. If you're feeling even more ambitious, you might try criss-crossing your arms when you jump—though don't be surprised if you get tangled up at first. Or try doing jump-rope jacks, in which you land with your feet apart on the first jump, then bring your feet together on the second jump: It's like jumping jacks, with the rope going all the time.

Jumping Rope Workouts

Beginner
Try 5 to 20 minutes of easy, two-footed jumping, paying attention to form. Start out with five 1-minute sessions between other interval activities. Work up to doing 1-minute jumping intervals for half the time. Do this combination three or four times a week.

Intermediate
Do 20 to 40 minutes of two-footed jumping—or alternating between one-footed and two-footed jumping—three or four times a week. Jump for 2-minute intervals, broken up by 3 minutes of another activity, so you are jumping two-thirds of the time.

Experienced
Alternate 3 minutes of rope skipping with 3 minutes of other activities for a total of 40 to 60 minutes.

POWER WALKING

Calories Burned
198 to 250 per mile

Body-Shaping Potential
Tones hips, thighs, buttocks, and abdominals

Here's what you can expect when you power walk regularly.

▶ If you are a regular walker but find that you have to walk long periods of time in order to burn as much fat as you want, then power walking will help you burn calories in less time.

▶ You will tone all the muscles in your lower body, including the gluteus, hamstrings, and quadriceps.

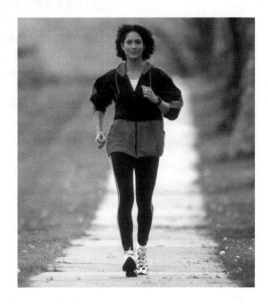

On Your Feet

"Try on as many walking shoes as possible before you buy a pair," recommends Carol Espel, a Walk Reebok master trainer and the executive fitness director of Equinox Fitness Clubs of New York. "You want to look for shoes that are lightweight and that breathe. (Look for mesh on the top or sides of the shoe.) The forefoot of the shoe should be flexible, so it bends fairly easily.

"A slanted, or beveled, heel makes it easier to walk with a heel-to-toe motion, which is one of the techniques of power walking. It puts less strain on your shin muscles, thus avoiding shin splints," adds Espel. "Ultimately, though, you have to find the shoe that's most comfortable for you."

Other Stuff You'll Need

While walking is the easiest form of exercise, power walking requires some technique. "It's

not just a matter of walking faster," says Espel.

"The difference between a 17-minute-per-mile 'health walker' and a 13-minute-per-mile 'power walker' is technique," notes Jeff Salvage, a Medford, New Jersey, junior national coordinator of U.S. Track and Field and a coach of many women of all levels and ages.

Here's what you'll need for your metamorphosis.

A trail or a treadmill. While there's nothing wrong with simply walking around your neighborhood, if you want to power walk, you'll want to know exactly how long your training ground is. To do that, you can map out a course that's 4 to 5 miles long, do laps on a high school track, or walk on a treadmill that records your pace and distance automatically. Each of these choices has its own benefits.

"Getting started can be as easy as walking through a park or your neighborhood, which is

Real Women
SHOW YOU HOW

Ruth Power Walks into Her Class Reunion 32 Pounds Thinner

New Year's Day 1993 was one of celebration for homemaker and mother Ruth Artz. Her second child, a son, was born, and she made a resolution. "I had a school reunion to go to in May," she says. "I was determined that, by the time the party rolled around, I would lose the 32 extra pounds left after my pregnancy."

At 5 feet 1 inch, Ruth weighed 113 pounds before her pregnancy. At high risk for pregnancy-related complications, she had to give up her twice-a-week aerobics. By the time she gave birth, she weighed more than 160 pounds; afterward, she weighed about 145.

"I went to see my aerobics teacher, Rosemary, and it turned out she had given up teaching," Ruth says. "Because her knees were bothering her, she was concentrating on the walking that she had been doing for 20 years, and she asked me to come along."

Ruth didn't think walking would be enough to get rid of the extra weight, but she tried it anyway. "Rosemary blew me away!" Ruth says. "She wasn't strolling. I couldn't even keep up with her at first. In fact, it took a while before I could reach her speed of 4 miles an hour."

Ruth noticed a difference in her body. "In about 5 months, I got down to about 115 pounds. I also made a real effort to watch what I ate and to drink a lot of water, and I used an abs workout video to flatten my abdominal muscles."

The next year, Ruth and Rosemary, who have remained walking partners until this day, began to compete in marathons. "Our normal walks are now 4½ miles per hour (a little over a 13-minute-per-mile pace), but because they have time limits, we try to walk 12-minute to 11½-minute miles when we do marathons," says Ruth. In fact, Ruth and Rosemary always aim to complete the 26.2-mile course in 6 hours or under.

At 35, Ruth walked the Walt Disney World Marathon, and her figure reflects her accomplishments. "I'm 103 pounds now, and I feel great," she says. "I'm in better shape now than I was in my early twenties. Having Rosemary to walk with really helped—I don't know what I would have done without her."

wonderful because of the scenery and varying terrain," says Espel. "Tracks are good because you can concentrate on technique and don't have to worry about traffic."

Breathing in the fresh air and letting the wind pass over your body is healthy. Treadmills, on the other hand, allow you to pinpoint your pace and distance, which is also very helpful in the beginning. Keep in mind, however, that you aren't getting the benefit of the fresh air.

Start with a warmup, advises Espel. Walk at a comfortable pace for about 5 minutes or until you break out in a light sweat. Then stretch your quadriceps, hips, hamstrings, and shins.

Water. If you're accustomed to waiting until you get home from your stroll to rehydrate, it's time to change. "You must carry a water bottle with you," says Espel. "Your power walks will be more intense than your old walks, so it's important to have water before, during, and after your workout." Drink at least a cup of water before starting out, a cup or more while you're walking, and still more water afterward.

If you don't want to carry the bottle in your hand, invest in a fanny pack or waist pack big enough to hold a bottle of water, or buy one that has a strap in which to place the bottle.

A progress log. Metamorphosing from a walker to a power walker means keeping track of your progress. "Your log doesn't have to be fancy or formal," says Espel. "Just write down when you walked, how far you went, how it felt, and how long it took you."

FAT BLASTER

Think about walking a marathon. Most of these events allow racewalkers to compete. You might start earlier than the runners, but you'll begin and finish the event in the same places. Believe it or not, professional racewalkers walk at a clip that isn't too far behind those of marathon runners. Most marathons are based on time, not gait, so you should ask what the time limit of the race is and decide whether it is reasonable for you.

Power Walking Workouts

Beginner
Using power-walking techniques, start to change the way you move during your walk. Bend your arms at a 90-degree angle, pump them, and try to walk heel-to-toe. Do this once or twice during your regular walks for a few weeks before moving on to the next level.

Intermediate
Start working intervals into your routine. For example, walk as fast as you can to a stop sign. Then give yourself time to recover (using a slower walk) before you start another interval. Do this three to five times during each walk for 20 to 30 seconds each for at least 4 or 5 weeks. It's an every-other-day workout.

Experienced
Start timing yourself and measuring your heart rate during your walks. Subtract your age from 220—that's your maximum heart rate. You should never work out at that rate; rather, aim for 60 to 90 percent of that number.

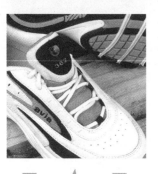 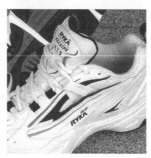 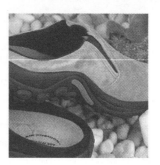 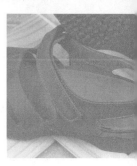

Walking
works
wonders

visit...

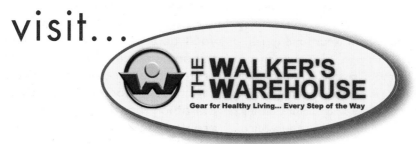

THE WALKER'S WAREHOUSE
Gear for Healthy Living... Every Step of the Way

and take a step
in the healthy direction

from path to pavement, we have the best selection in footwear and so much mor

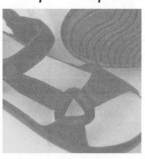 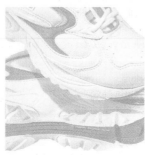 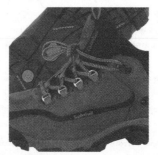 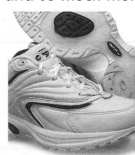

45-Day Guarantee on all Products • Superior Customer Service

ROWING

Calories Burned

240 to 360 per half-hour

Body-Shaping Potential

Tones the entire body, especially the muscles of the thighs, buttocks, abdominals, back, and arms

Here's what you can expect when you row regularly.

▶ You'll burn calories galore, because you're using all four limbs while your heart works—which uses up more calories than lower-body exercise alone, says J. Zack Barksdale, an exercise physiologist at the Cooper Aerobics Center in Dallas.

▶ You'll develop strong, toned abdominals, because you'll contract your abdominal muscles when you're rowing. When you contract your abdominal muscles consistently, they get stronger. When a woman's muscles get stronger, they get toned and develop more shape, even though they don't get bigger. Your legs and butt do a tremendous amount of work, so they also grow lean and strong.

▶ As a bonus, you'll tone and strengthen your upper arms, an added trouble spot for many women as they reach midlife.

On Your Feet

For all practical purposes, most women who want to row for exercise just buy rowing machines and put them to work in their living rooms, basements, or other workout space. That doesn't mean you should row in just any footwear. Wear low-cut sneakers to allow range of motion in your ankles, says Holly Metcalf, president and founder of Row as One Institute, a rowing school and camp for women located in South Hadley,

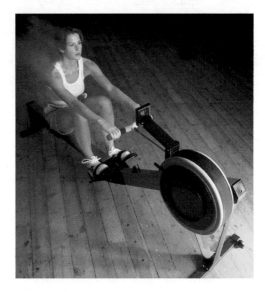

Massachusetts. She also recommends wearing tights and an exercise top. "Loose clothes, such as shorts and T-shirts, can get caught in the machine and won't allow you to move as smoothly."

Other Stuff You'll Need

If you're like a lot of women, chances are you—or someone in your family—already have an indoor rower stashed somewhere in the garage or basement. If it's more than a couple of years old, you may want to consider buying new equipment or using a rower at a gym or fitness club, says Barksdale. Check to make sure that your older rower has not become creaky or damaged over the years. If so, it may need a little oil to return to working order, he adds.

Unless your shoulders are very strong, you may be better off not using an older rower at all. Many rowers made in the 1980s feature two "oars" that move independently of one another (rather than a pulley), along with piston-driven resistance. Both features can make rowing potentially stressful on the shoulders and rotator cuffs, Barksdale cautions.

Here's what to look for.

Sturdy equipment with an ample seat and adjustable footpads. The only parts of your body that touch the rower are your hands, feet, and backside. The footpads should be easy to adjust for foot size. And when you row, the equipment should remain steady and secure on the floor.

If you're big-bottomed, pay special attention to how you fit in the saddle. Your backside must fit comfortably in the seat. Also, a big tummy may interfere with your range of motion and force you to hold your legs out to your sides, causing stress on the ligaments of your knees. Or you may round your back while rowing, which could potentially lead to back problems. If you have quite a bit of weight to lose, you may have to wait until your tummy and backside shrink to work rowing into your shape-up program, says Barksdale. If you're very overweight, you could also consider starting on a recumbent, he says.

Air or water resistance. Both air and water resistance give a smoother ride than the older piston-resistance machines, and they more closely simulate the outdoor rowing experience. The WaterRower actually uses a water flywheel for resistance, so it very closely simulates outdoor rowing on water. The water level can be adjusted to increase or decrease the resistance. The rhythm and adjustable wind resistance of the Concept II (found in most gyms) also mimic the feeling of river rowing. Both models are available through mail order.

Space. Indoor rowers are long—at least 6 feet. So if you're buying equipment, you'll need to make sure that you have enough room for it at home.

FAT BLASTER

If rowing inspires you to take to the water, call a local college or high school to see if they have a rowing coach. He or she will probably know of a women's masters team (geared toward women in their forties or older) in your area—assuming you live near a major lake or river. This is a major commitment: Most teams practice either during the early morning or early evening. How often depends on their training and racing schedule. But it's practically guaranteed to help you get in shape.

Rowing Workouts

Beginner	Intermediate	Experienced
Row for 20 minutes at least twice a week. Keep the resistance light, but not so light that momentum moves you.	Row hard for 30 seconds, then easy for 30 seconds. Try to do 20 to 40 minutes at least three times a week.	Warm up for 5 to 10 minutes, then keep a steady, high-intensity pace going for 40 to 60 minutes. Do not bend your knees past a 90-degree angle. Cool down. Repeat 4 or 5 days a week.

SPINNING

Calories Burned
About 535 per 45-minute class

Body-Shaping Potential
Trims the butt and thighs, tones the abdominal muscles

Here's what you can expect when you spin regularly.

▶ You'll burn 600 to 800 calories an hour—about as much as rowing on a machine at race pace.

▶ You'll tone your entire lower body, especially your butt and the front of your thighs.

▶ If you do a lot of standing and sitting intervals (known as jumps), you'll strengthen your abdominal muscles.

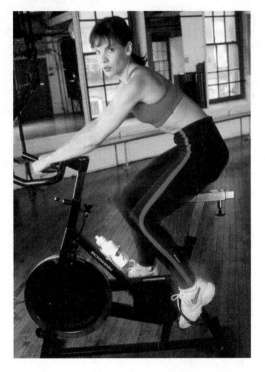

On Your Feet

Like the pedals on traditional racing bikes, Spinning bike pedals consist of a "cage," which holds your sneakered foot steady, and a "lock" for bike shoes. "Locking your foot into the pedal helps you move your legs more smoothly," explains Ron Crawford, a certified Spinning instructor from Niles, Ohio. "But not everyone likes the feel of bike shoes." Most bike pedal manufacturers have a universal lock, which means that most bike shoes will fit into any bike pedal, Spinning or otherwise.

Other Stuff You'll Need

Very few people purchase their own Spinning bikes because so much of the sport's appeal is its group atmosphere. So chances are you'll join a class. If you do, here's what Deborah Gallagher, a certified personal trainer and certified Spinning instructor in Vacaville, California, suggests you bring along.

Water. Spinning bikes include built-in water-bottle holders for a very good reason—you're going to need to stay hydrated during the class. Most of the holders will fit a small bottle of water—preferably one with a pop-up spout, so you don't have to interrupt your ride to open up your bottle.

A towel. You'll need a small hand towel not only to sop up the sweat from your forehead but also to wipe down your bike before someone else gets ready to use it.

Bike shorts (maybe). Like riding any bike, Spinning can irritate a tender tush (or

Real Women
SHOW YOU HOW

Denise Got Back into a Size 8

Denise Carissimo, director of admissions at a business college, was starting to feel stagnant in her life. At just 34 years old, she felt as if she had peaked. Plus, she was gaining weight—and getting bottom-heavy.

"I normally wore a size 8," says Denise. "But I was stuffing myself into my size 10 clothes. I really should have been wearing a 12."

Then she tried her first Spinning class.

"I was addicted immediately," Denise says. "I began Spinning three times a week for 40 minutes each. The intensity level was great. It made me feel so alive and excited. And even though I didn't change the way I was eating, I was dropping inches like crazy!"

Denise noticed the difference within 2 to 3 months. "My bottom half is trimmed down, and I feel better. My waist is tiny. Even my calves look slimmer."

Those inches made all the difference in the way Denise's clothes fit. She began to comfortably wear her old size 8 clothing again. "I still weigh the same amount, but you would never know it from the way I look."

other sensitive spots). "Bike shorts have extra padding in the butt to cushion you," says Gallagher. "They're available at most sporting goods stores."

A gel seat. Some gyms provide bike seats filled with gel, while others expect you to bring your own. "Available at sporting goods stores, gel seats have a lot more give than a traditional bike seat," notes Gallagher. "Some people prefer gel seats to bike shorts—especially if you don't look great in close-fitting shorts or can't find them in your size."

Spinning Workouts

Beginner	Intermediate	Experienced
Take Begin to Spin classes twice a week, with no jumping allowed. Keep this schedule consistent for 4 to 6 weeks.	Move on to three classes per week. To work your legs, work out at a slightly higher pedaling speed.	After 2 to 3 months of steady riding (three times a week), include jumping and other intense moves like sprinting (high-speed pedaling at light to moderate resistance).

STATIONARY CYCLING

Calories Burned
130 to 330 per half-hour

Body-Shaping Potential
Tones the leg and butt muscles

Here's what you can expect when you use a stationary cycle regularly.

▶ You'll burn about 5 calories every minute while you exercise. That's a lot more than the usual 1 calorie per minute that you burn when you're doing other daily activities.

▶ You'll develop and strengthen the gluteal muscles in your buttocks, the quadriceps at the front of your thighs, and the hamstrings in the back of your thighs.

▶ There's no impact from your upper-body weight, so you can tone your butt and thigh muscles without putting any stress on your leg joints.

What You'll Need

A good, new home bike costs a minimum of $350. But if that's more than you would like to pay, post a notice or ad for used bikes and see what kind of response you get. You may be able to get a used bike for much less than a similar new model.

Whatever you do, be sure to sit on the bike and pedal for a while to see how comfortable it is for you. "Wear your gym clothes, including your sneakers," says Edmund Burke, Ph.D., professor of exercise science at the University of Colorado in Colorado Springs. "If it doesn't feel right, try another model."

Whether you're buying new or used, here's what to consider.

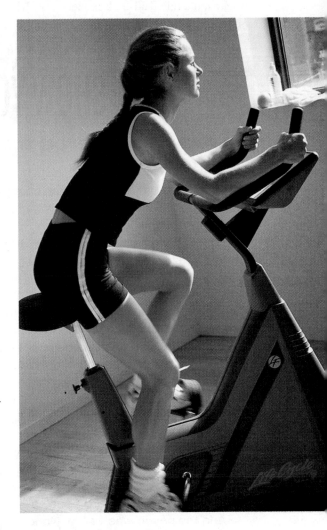

Upright or recumbent. Traditional upright bikes aren't designed for women and overweight people, in general, because the seats aren't wide enough. And an upright can spell torture if you have lower-back pain. Before you write a check, be sure to try out a recumbent bike, which has a bucket-shaped seat that supports your back. Or you might like something in-between an upright and a fully laid-back model—called a semirecumbent.

The right fit. First of all, you should be able to sit up straight on the bike even when you are pedaling full speed. This isn't a bike for the Tour de France, where you have

Real Women
SHOW YOU HOW

Nancy Discovered the Permanent Route to Weight Loss

Nancy Allen's father died when she was 37. The loss hurt—as she knew it would. So much, in fact, that it seemed as though she stopped doing anything for a while.

"My dad died around Christmas, and I just became a lump for about 4 months," she says. "Because I was getting older, this change of pace led to a pretty fast weight gain. I'm only 5 feet 3 inches tall, and I ended up being somewhere around a size 12."

After 4 months of inactivity, Nancy decided she'd had enough with languishing on the couch. On April 4—she remembers the exact date—she started exercising on the recumbent stationary bike that had been sitting in the corner of her living room for some time.

The months of inactivity had taken their toll, however. "I could only do about 3 minutes," she recalls. But when she got off, the impact of that little spurt of exercise surprised her. "I felt so much better!"

Within about a week, Nancy was pedaling up to 5 minutes every day. From there, she advanced rapidly until she could do about 15 minutes daily. Four years later, at the age of 41, Nancy is still doing a steady routine of 30 to 45 minutes daily. "My target heart rate is 23 beats per 10 seconds. I'm usually puffing pretty hard," she says.

And the payoff was visible. Nancy went from a size 12 to a size 5. "My waist was somewhere around 33 to 34 inches, and now it is 26 inches," she says. "I have no saddlebags anymore, and my butt is gravity-defying."

She credits the almost-forgotten stationary cycle and the human spirit that just wouldn't quit with starting it all. "All the equipment in the world won't help without the determination to use it," she adds.

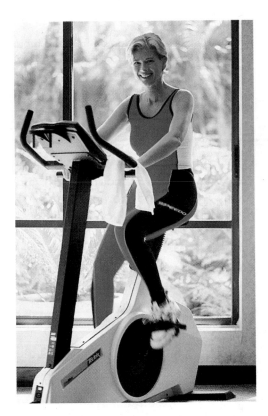

toes of your foot below the knee. If you cannot see your toes, then you are too far forward. Sitting too far forward puts enormous stress on the kneecap. After you have made all the necessary seat adjustments, then see whether the handlebars are still at a comfortable level. If not, adjust them, too.

The same criteria apply to a recumbent bike. You should be able to move the seat forward or back, up or down. When it is in the correct position, your extended leg should be slightly bent at the knee.

A gel seat. Though you may think your hips and butt are well-padded, an ordinary bicycle seat can feel like an abrasive torture device after many miles of spinning. If you're getting a brand-new bike, ask the salesperson if you can have a softer gel seat instead of the standard-issue seat. If you're getting a used bike, you can still find a gel seat at most bicycle or exercise equipment stores.

Upper-body exercise handles. Rather than having normal stationary handlebars, some bikes have handles that you can push and pull, so you'll get some upper-body exercise while your lower limbs are also going full steam ahead. You might enjoy the extra upper-body flex, but movable handles don't increase calorie burning very much. And they are an extra expense. So if you don't think you'll use that feature, skip it and stick to the pedal-only version.

Resistance. On some stationary bikes, resistance is created by a brake pad applying steady pressure. Others use electromagnetic resistance or a flywheel. The type of resistance might affect the feel of the bike, but otherwise, there is no particular advantage to any of them. You do want to be able to adjust the resistance

to crouch over the handlebars and look like a flying bullet. If you need to hunch over to reach the handlebars, then the bike isn't the right size for you.

Adjustability. No bike is made-to-order, so you need to be able to make adjustments, explains Cyndi Ford, an exercise physiologist at the Cooper Institute for Aerobics Research in Dallas. When you're trying out the bike, make sure that you can move the seat up or down to the right position. When you're seated on an upright bike, your hips should be square on the saddle. At the bottom of the downstroke, with your foot rested firmly on the lower pedal, the extended leg should be slightly bent at the knee. Also, look straight down and see whether you can see the so that you can vary the intensity of your workouts.

Electronics. Some bikes have elaborate programs—along with heart-rate monitors and other devices—to help you measure many different variables. With some, you can race against a computerized competitor. If you like these features and they keep you more challenged, you might want to opt for them. But they don't affect the operation of the bike or the slimming and trimming benefits you get from it.

Some other useful hints:

Padded bike shorts. The shorts worn by bicyclists have a built-in chafing-prevention device. It's called extra padding. Strategically sewn into the crotch and inner-thigh region of the shorts, the padding can make indoor as well as outdoor riding more comfortable.

Repairs. Find out how, and where, you can get the bike fixed if something goes wrong. When equipment breaks, workouts come to a standstill.

FAT BLASTER

Ride the Tour de France in your living room. A number of companies sell bike ride videos that you can watch while you are exercising. You can tour the south of France or national parks while you pedal or even take part in famous road races. These tapes are often available wherever exercise videos are sold.

Stationary Cycling Workouts

Beginner

Progressive intervals. Over a 22-minute period, intersperse slow-paced, low-intensity riding with short, higher-intensity spurts. Ride at a slow pace and low intensity for 5 minutes, then pedal for 30 seconds at higher intensity. Keep alternating, but end up with some slow pedaling to cool down.

Intermediate

Pyramid workout. Ride for 10 minutes at high intensity, then follow with 2 minutes of low-intensity riding. Then do 8 minutes at a level of intensity that's even higher than the first 10 minutes—followed by another 2-minute, low-intensity interlude. Each increasingly harder interval should be 2 minutes shorter than the one before, but keep on increasing the intensity—and always insert a 2-minute interval to cool down. The whole routine should take about 40 minutes. Then give yourself some slow pedaling at the end to finish off.

Experienced

Hill training. If you want to test your maximum capacity, plan on riding for a certain amount of time—say, 40 minutes—and use progressively higher resistance throughout the ride. Increase the resistance every 3 to 4 minutes to increase the intensity of your workout. When you are halfway through the session, decrease the resistance at regular intervals over the same amount of time.

STEP AEROBICS

Calories Burned
Approximately 300 per half-hour using a 6-inch step

Body-Shaping Potential
Works the entire lower body—hips, thighs, and buttocks

Here's what you can expect when you do step aerobics regularly.

▶ You will burn lots of fat, since step aerobics is a high-intensity exercise.

▶ You'll tone and shape the muscles in your lower body, especially your butt, thighs, and calves.

▶ If you concentrate on keeping your abdominals contracted while you step, you'll tone and strengthen your abdominal muscles.

On Your Feet

You'll want support while you do your step aerobics routine, so a good pair of aerobic shoes is your best bet. Look for flexible shoes that have plenty of cushioning and arch support on the bottom, recommends Tamilee Webb, the choreographer of numerous step videos and author of *The Step Up Fitness Workout*, who lives in San Diego. Some women prefer higher-cut shoes that give their ankles extra support.

Other Stuff You'll Need

Once you've laced up your shoes, you'll need a step bench, a low and wide platform with graduated risers, so you can increase step height as you become more experienced at step aerobics. Some risers are attached to the step and simply fold

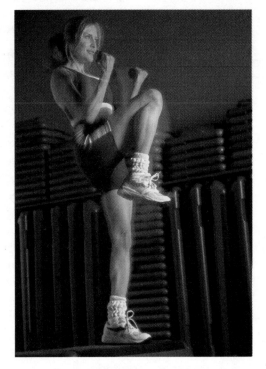

under it when you want to change the step height.

Here's what to look for in a step bench, according to Webb.

Sturdy construction. Because you'll be stepping up and down on the bench, it should feel as solid as any step you would climb in your house. Likewise, any risers that come with the step should also be solid and not wobble at all as you go up and down the bench.

A step that is wide and long enough. You need plenty of room for both of your feet on the bench. Some choreography won't work with a narrow step, so if the step bench is too narrow, it's not a good buy. You should also be able to take at least one step out to the side while you're on the bench. The ideal

Real Women
SHOW YOU HOW

Beth Burned Off 25 Pounds

Beth Mendelson, age 41, loves her three boys—she would do anything for them. What she doesn't like is *looking* like somebody's mom. Step aerobics changed all that.

The turning point was when Beth went to a restaurant with some friends. As they passed through the bar, "none of the men looked at me at all," she says. "I was 35 at the time, but I looked a lot older."

At 5 feet 1 and 140 pounds, Beth decided to do something. "I had always been intimidated by traditional aerobics classes because I felt klutzy," she says. "But I figured I'd be okay exercising in my own home. So I went to the library and rented some aerobics tapes. But I still didn't like aerobics."

Then someone loaned Beth a step bench and step aerobics tape. "I loved it!" she says. "It was easy for me to build my confidence. Because the music is slower, my feet and brain work better with step."

Beth started with a beginner tape by Kathy Smith and then went on to Gin Miller's Reebok series. She loves tapes by Cathe Friedrich, one of the toughest instructors around. "I've found that I'm always able to pick up the choreography after using one tape just a few times," Beth says. "When I get a new tape, I really have to concentrate when I first use it; as I become more comfortable with it, I'm able to focus more on giving my body a tough workout instead of memorizing the new moves."

Step aerobics has really paid off for Beth. She now weighs about 115 pounds. "My thighs are slimmer, firmer, and much more muscular," she notes. "But, more than that, I feel like I look good now. I absolutely don't think I look my age."

step is 2 feet wide and 3 feet long. You can buy shorter (and cheaper) step benches, but the longer and wider the bench is, the more intense you'll be able to make your workouts.

Getting Started

Step aerobics is a high-intensity exercise, so you'll want to begin your workout routine slowly. Experts recommend videotapes specifically geared toward beginners (such as those offered by instructors such as Gin Miller, Tamilee Webb, or Kathy Smith, for example). Once you select a tape, here's how to use it.

First, master the legs, then add your arms. When you're first learning to perform step aerobics, don't worry about moving your arms, even if the instructor on the workout tape is mixing her arms into the patterns. Instead, concentrate on getting the foot patterns down and feeling comfortable using the platform, says Miller.

The basic step pattern goes "up-up, down-down," up with the right foot, up with the left foot, down with the right foot, down with the left foot. "It's just like the way a child first learns to climb a staircase," says Webb. "The most important thing to remember is that you have to place your whole foot on the step, not just your toes and not just the ball of your foot."

When you're ready, begin to incorporate the arm movements into your routine. Continuous arm movements increase your heart rate, and thus the number of calories you burn, by up to 10 percent.

Forget the hand weights. Hand weights can limit movement, and they can also cause pain and fatigue in your shoulders when used for long periods of time, cautions Webb.

Limit yourself to no more than four step workouts a week. Studies have shown that doing step aerobics more than four times a week markedly increases the chance of injury. So be happy that it's a high-intensity workout that will burn tons of calories in a very short amount of time.

Increase the step height very gradually. The Reebok stepping platform—considered a "benchmark"-size step by experts—is 6 inches high. You can adjust the height by 2 inches at a time to make the advanced step bench a total height of up to 10 inches. When you feel comfortable doing your step routine at the lowest height, add height 2 inches at a time, until your leg reaches a 60-degree angle or a comfortable step height.

FAT BLASTER

Think you have all the step possibilities down pat? Then crank up your stereo and choreograph your own workout, using a combination of low-, moderate-, and high-intensity moves.

Step Aerobics Workouts

Beginner	Intermediate	Experienced
Perform a 30-minute workout that begins with an 8-minute warmup and ends with a 5-minute cooldown. Start by doing this twice a week for 3 weeks to 1 month.	Increase one of three things: intensity (use more difficult moves and/or more arm combinations), duration (work out for a total of 40 to 50 minutes), or the number of times you exercise (try three or four times a week). Don't increase all three at once, and keep switching things around for a month to 6 weeks.	Add the hard moves, like lunges. Don't work out for longer than 60 minutes, or more often than four times per week.

STEPPING AND STAIRCLIMBING MACHINES

Calories Burned
250 to 350 per half-hour

Body-Shaping Potential
Tones butt, thighs, hips, and calves

Repeatedly raising and lowering your body with either a stepper or stairclimber uses all of the large muscles in your hips, butt, thighs, and lower legs. As a result, stepping combines calorie burning (which uses fat as energy, so it comes off your body) with lower-body sculpting.

Here's what you can expect when you use a stepper regularly.

▶ You'll tone and strengthen your butt and thigh muscles, leaving you with a smaller butt and leaner thighs.

▶ You'll develop shapelier calf muscles.

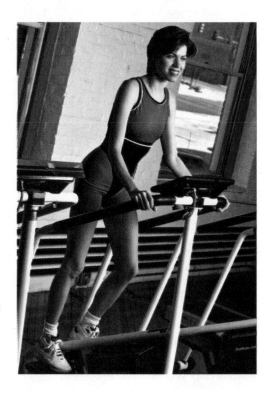

Other Stuff You'll Need

Any type of athletic shoe or comfortable sneaker will work on a step machine, so you don't have to go out and buy elaborate footwear.

You'll find steppers or stairclimbers in most gyms, so you don't necessarily have to buy one—unless you want to. Like other forms of exercise equipment, such as treadmills and weight machines, step machines are convenient, but the good ones can run you some money.

Here are some questions to ask and features to think about when you're considering a step machine at a gym or shopping for a home model.

Is it sturdy? The equipment should be able to support your weight easily and remain steady even while you're in motion, says Carla Sottovia, assistant fitness director at the Cooper Fitness Center in Dallas. The more expensive machines are usually sturdier and a better buy for people who have a significant amount of weight to lose.

Is it the right size? Every step machine has a prescribed range of distance that the footpad can travel as you step. Some ranges are wider than others. It should be easy for you to stay in the midrange, or "sweet spot," of the step length. Likewise, the footpads should be big

Real Women
SHOW YOU HOW

Glenda Stepped Away from 40 Pounds

At one point, Glenda Holmes was at her highest weight ever—293 pounds. A 46-year-old kindergarten teacher, Glenda talked to her cousin Jim, who wanted to help her find a way to exercise. He suggested a step machine and offered to buy one for her.

They didn't talk about it again until just before Christmas, when Jim called to tell her someone would be calling to make delivery arrangements. "I had a cold around the holidays, so I didn't get on the machine until after the New Year," says Glenda. "The first time I got on it, I could only do 2 minutes with the machine set at the lowest intensity.

"I put the step machine in my dining room, so I'd have to walk past it every day," says Glenda. "I also decided that I would work out in the morning while listening to National Public Radio. That way, I knew I'd get it done early in the day before other responsibilities would get in my way."

This level-headed and realistic approach worked. Glenda lost over 40 pounds the first year and dropped two dress sizes. "My legs firmed up, and my butt, I must say, developed a perkier, more lifted look," she adds.

Glenda worked up to 25 minutes at a time at a higher intensity on her step machine. "I do 20 minutes on the manual program, then I do the last 5 minutes on a higher-intensity program, before finishing with a thorough cooldown lasting 5 to 6 minutes," she says. "And I continue to get better and better at it."

enough to hold your entire foot with room to spare. Try each machine to see which one feels most comfortable to you, suggests Sottovia.

How does it work? There are two different kinds of step machine designs, dependent and independent. If you push down on one step of a dependent machine, the other step will rise, creating greater stress on the knee joint. Independent steps aren't connected by anything and involve more natural and less stressful movement, says Cedric X. Bryant,

Ph.D., senior vice president of research and development/sports medicine at the StairMaster Corporation in Kirkland, Washington.

Most brands of step machines offer display monitors with manual or programmed features that set and measure the time and intensity of your effort. The programs also help you check your progress and guide you through a variety of workouts. You don't need an elaborately programmed unit to get a good workout, though, says Dr. Bryant. Choose a machine based on how the equipment moves as you exercise, not the display features, he says.

What type of resistance does it use? Experts recommend buying either hydraulic, cable, or chain steppers. Be careful, though, since hydraulic machines (which are less expensive) use oil, which can leak onto home carpeting. Leading brands of steppers include StairMaster, Tunturi, VersaClimber, and Tectrix.

Getting Started

Stepping might look as easy as marching, but stepping improperly can cost you 75 calories per workout. Bad form can also contribute to uncomfortable aches and pains during and after your workout. To step safely and effectively, you have to do it right. Here's how.

Warm up. As with any exercise, a good rule for stepping is "start slow, stop gradually," says Sottovia. "Warm up for 5 minutes with smaller steps on a low resistance level, then move into your workout with longer steps at a higher resistance. Slow down again at the end, and make sure you stretch your leg muscles afterward."

Don't lean on the rails. "When people lean, they tend to do about 20 to 25 percent less work than the machine credits them for, because they aren't using their full body weight when they step," says Dr. Bryant. "If you're working so hard that you have to lean on the machine, lower the stepping speed. Your hands should rest lightly, if at all, on the handlebars."

Slow down. Stepping quickly doesn't mean you'll burn more calories. It's the force of your leg working against the step, not how fast you step, that determines the value of the workout. Your steps should cover the middle range of the whole length of the step, and your speed should be steady, not fast or choppy, according to Dr. Bryant.

FAT BLASTER

If you like the feel of using a stepper but wish your upper body could get a workout, too, look into using a vertical climbing machine, such as the VersaClimber by Heart Rate. It's a lot like climbing a stationary ladder, and because you work your arms and legs in full range of motion, you'll burn lots of calories.

Stepping Workouts

Beginner	Intermediate	Experienced
Start with 5 minutes at the lowest level you feel comfortable with, every day, if possible. Work your way up to 20 minutes at this intensity.	Once you can do 20 minutes of exercise every day, cut down on frequency, but increase intensity. Exercise for 2 days on and 1 day off, raising the intensity level every few workouts. Aim for 20 minutes, three or four times per week.	Alternate between high and moderate intensity: For every minute of high-intensity exercise, do 2 minutes of moderate-intensity work. Continue for 20 minutes, three or four times a week.

SWIMMING

Calories Burned

249 to 351 per half-hour, depending on the stroke and speed

Body-Shaping Potential

High-calorie burning; tones the legs, hips, torso, arms, back, and chest

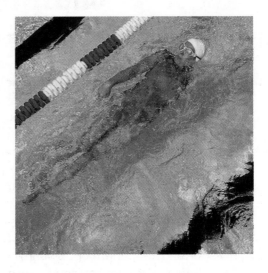

Here's what you can expect when you swim regularly.

▶ You'll burn as many calories as running, without stressing your knees or bones.

▶ You'll tone your abdomen and hips.

▶ You'll tone and strengthen your legs. As a bonus, you'll also firm up your chest and upper arms.

Other Stuff You'll Need

Let's start with the big item.

A pool. Maybe you'll be swimming in a lake or the ocean. But most women who swim regularly are probably doing laps at their local pool or YWCA.

A bathing suit. If you're like a lot of women, the thought of wearing a swimsuit in public makes you cringe. "It's just a matter of getting from the edge of the pool into the water," says Jane Katz, Ed.D., professor of health and physical education at the John Jay College of Criminal Justice of the City University of New York in New York City. "Once you're in there, no one can see what you look like."

That said, Dr. Katz advises women who swim for exercise to buy a racing suit designed and produced by sportswear companies. "Shop at a sporting goods store first, rather than a department store," she says. "You're not looking for something to lounge in, but rather something that will hold your body in place and keep you streamlined in the water." For exercise swimming, she advises women to stay away from suits with skirts or other added layers of fabric.

Fortunately, the traditional racer-back suit, which is available in almost all sizes, is flattering to almost every figure, since it covers your backside and upper thighs more adequately than fashion swimsuits that are cut high on the thigh. For large-breasted women, Dr. Katz recommends fitness swimsuits with support. "You can purchase these at specialty fitness stores where swimsuits are geared to accommodate your form."

Finally, Dr. Katz has one other piece of advice for the bathing-suit shy: "Swim at a facility that's not too high-brow. More expensive clubs tend to be more looks-oriented, but your local Y caters to every type of body."

Real Women
SHOW YOU HOW

Gigi Lost 160 Pounds in the Pool

One phone call really can change a woman's life. "I remember the nurse at my doctor's office called to tell me that my cholesterol was slightly elevated," says Gigi Carnes, 39, a curator. "When I asked her what that meant, she actually started to yell at me. 'You need to eat better!' she said. 'You need to lose weight!'"

Gigi says she couldn't deny that she had a problem: She weighed 310 pounds and wore a size 28.

At just about the same time, a nearby swim club opened up in May for the season. So Gigi got into her bathing suit and started swimming. She swam 5 days a week and sometimes 6 in the hot days of summer. "The weight just rolled off me," she says. "By July, I needed to tie a cord around my shorts to keep them up. Swimming was obviously making a difference." Less than a year after starting to swim regularly, Gigi was 160 pounds lighter.

Goggles. To minimize levels of harmful bacteria, pool water must contain a certain amount of chlorine and other disinfecting chemicals that can irritate your eyes, so you need goggles. They're a must for swimming laps, says Dr. Katz, because they allow you to see the lane markers along the bottom of the pool. Goggles aren't expensive; pick up a pair at a specialty fitness store where someone can help you choose the best-fitting ones. For beginning swimmers, Dr. Katz recommends goggles with good peripheral vision and padding around the rim of the eyepiece. You should feel light suction around the eyes—just enough to keep water out.

A bathing cap. Public pools sometimes require women (and sometimes men) to wear a bathing cap. Wearing a cap also helps to protect your hair from chemicals in the pool water, which can dry or discolor your hair. And if your hair is long, a cap keeps it from becoming tangled while you swim. Look for something sleek and simple at a specialty fitness store. A silicone bathing cap is best because it doesn't pull your hair as much as other materials do, explains Dr. Katz.

Getting Started

"Swimming for exercise is not the same as taking a dip when you're hot and want to cool off after a day in the sun," points out Dr. Katz. "You have to swim at a consistent pace for at least 20 minutes in order to get your heart pumping and your fat burning."

Crawl first. Unless you're proficient in another stroke (breast, back, side, or butterfly), you'll probably want to do the crawl, which is sometimes called freestyle swimming. Before you attempt to learn several different strokes, simply work on being able to consistently do a crawl for 10 minutes at a time, suggests Dr. Katz.

Learn to roll. Sure, swimming looks as if your arms and legs are providing all the power. But the real source of a swimmer's power comes from the hips and trunk. "Efficient swimmers are always in a rolling motion," says Dr. Katz. "They're never still in the water." The key is to move from your hips, turning your head to one side to breathe as the opposite arm comes out of the water, then starting to roll toward the other side for your next breath and its matching stroke.

Turn your head and inhale. If you haven't swum laps for a long time, you may feel awkward trying to pace your breaths. When you breathe, turn your whole head along with your body toward one side. Your mouth will lift slightly out of the water for an inhalation. As your body rolls back into a straight line, you'll slowly blow bubbles as you exhale into the water. Continue your body roll to the other side, turning your mouth out of the water on the other side for your next inhalation. Alternating breathing in this way helps to balance your stroke, says Dr. Katz. When you become a proficient swimmer, alternate breathing sides every third pull.

Lead with your head, not your chin. Your head, not your chin, should lead the way down the lane, says Dr. Katz. You want your body in one streamlined position so that you're looking toward the floor of the pool. Don't worry about hitting the wall—when you see the end of the black line in your lane, start to make your turn, and swim back down the lane.

FAT BLASTER

Flip onto your back. A major calorie burner (345 calories per half-hour if you weigh 150 pounds), the backstroke is a wonderful complement to the crawl. If you don't like to keep your face in the water, you'll like this stroke.

Swimming Workouts

Beginner

Swim freestyle laps for a total of 100 to 300 yards every other day or at least three times a week for 1 to 2 months. If you have to stop in between laps at first, that's okay. Work up to swimming nonstop for 10 minutes. If you use fins, you'll burn more calories.

Intermediate

Swim 350 to 550 yards in about 15 minutes without stopping, at least three times a week for 2 months.

Experienced

Swim 600 yards (24 laps in a 25-yard pool) to 880 yards at a time without stopping, three times a week. Mix and match your strokes, if you want. This should take about 30 minutes.

TENNIS

Calories Burned

475 an hour in a highly competitive match

Body-Shaping Potential

Tones the gluteus, quadriceps, hamstrings, and calf muscles

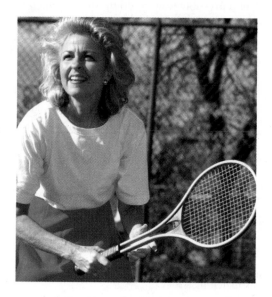

Whichever arm you use primarily to play tennis will become stronger and shapelier as a result of playing the game, but this sport primarily provides a lower-body workout. If you play tennis regularly:

▶ Your gluteus, quadriceps, hamstrings, and calf muscles will all get a good workout from the quick starts and stops and lateral movements required in tennis.

On Your Feet

Wearing the right shoes is important in tennis. Running shoes and cross-trainers are not designed for the game's constant lateral movement, says Paul van der Sommen, owner and tennis instructor at the Oneonta Tennis Club in Oneonta, New York. "If you wear tennis shoes, you'll have less risk of ankle injury when playing."

Here's what to look for, according to Barrett Bugg, exercise science specialist for the U.S. Tennis Association, based in Key Biscayne, Florida.

Good arch support. A shoe that's well-designed for racket sports will have good support for the arch and be well-padded at the ball of the foot, where you exert the most pressure. If the arch supports feel too high, try another style.

Toe room. There should be enough room in the toebox to move your toes and avoid blisters. That means no more than ¼ inch between the toes and the toebox or front of the shoe. The toebox is subject to the most wear and tear during tennis, so make sure it's made of leather or rubber, not fabric, which will wear out faster.

Wide soles. The outsole, or bottom, of the shoe should be wider than the upper—the part of the shoe above the sole. Otherwise, you won't be getting enough lateral support as you move from side to side on the court. Look for a midsole made of ethyl vinyl acetate (EVA) or polyurethane. Some shoes have air or gel within the midsole. Press the shoe. The midsole should give a bit. The insole, or interior, of the shoe should be made of fabric that will breathe and control moisture.

The right size. Buy tennis shoes that are one-half size larger than your regular shoe size, so they can accommodate heavy tennis socks.

Thick socks. Look for thick socks in moisture-wicking fabric or synthetic/cotton blends that provide extra cushioning to absorb shocks and prevent blisters. Ankle-length socks are best; low-cut socks—even with pom-poms at the heel—tend to creep back into tennis shoes. Some players wear two pairs of socks to minimize blisters and maximize moisture absorption and cushioning, Bugg adds.

Other Stuff You'll Need

Tennis doesn't require much equipment. Here's what you'll need.

The right racket. Beginners should buy a lightweight, oversize racket, which will improve their chances of making contact with the ball, says Jim Coyne, director of tennis at the Claremont Resort in Berkeley, California. If your racket's too heavy, your arm will get tired. But if it's too light, you'll be waving it like a wand, not learning proper strokes.

Look for a racket with midlevel string tension, to absorb impact but provide power. As for grip, a finger's width should separate the tip of your middle finger from the crease at the base of your thumb as you grasp the handle.

If you plan to play at a club, ask at the pro shop if you can rent or borrow a racket for the

Real Women
SHOW YOU HOW

Ronda Lost Weight—And Mellowed Out

When Ronda Sorensen took up tennis, it wasn't exercise she craved. It was adult conversation. Ronda had quit her job to stay home with her two young children, and she missed talking to other grown-ups during the day.

Playing tennis solved the problem, and it offered Ronda an added benefit. After playing regularly, she lost about 10 pounds. "People always say I look leaner," says Sorensen, 38. "And I think I'm stronger, too."

Ronda also believes in the mental magic of tennis. "If you've had a bad day, like with your kids, it's much better to be batting around a bunch of balls than getting angry with your children. When I come home from playing tennis, I'm Mellow Mom."

Ronda plays three sets of tennis 3 or 4 days a week, typically spending 1½ to 2 hours each day on the court. She even competed in an amateur tournament in Florida, which further helped to keep her in shape.

"I've seen myself improve, and I want to get better," Sorensen says. "I just love the game."

day and see if it feels like a model you might want to buy.

Fresh balls. All tennis balls are created equal, says van der Sommen. So if you can buy a can cheaper at a discount store, do so. Balls last longer in warmer climates. If it's summer or you live someplace like Florida where the weather is warm year-round, you can use the same balls two or three times, he says. If it's cold outside, they lose their bounce after play—use the balls only once.

Tennis attire. Some tennis clubs have a dress code requiring women to wear a skirt or a dress when playing tennis and men to wear a collared shirt. Others permit you to wear shorts. Some allow only all-white attire, or light colors. Of course, if you're playing on a public court—say, at a local community park or high school—you can wear what you please.

Whatever you wear should be comfortable, but not baggy or too snug. If you wear clothing that's too large, the excess fabric may slow you down. Clothing that's too tight can restrict your movements and not allow your skin to breathe. If you wear shorts instead of a tennis skirt, look for wide legs and side vents, to give you freedom of movement. Wear a sports bra to control bounce and support your breasts comfortably during play.

Cotton fabric is traditional for tennis, but it's best when blended with synthetics like Lycra or Supplex, which help clothing keep its shape longer and resist wrinkling.

Getting Started

You needn't be rich or competitive to enjoy tennis. "It's a wonderful sport to learn if the emphasis is not on winning," notes van der Sommen. Here are some tips on getting started.

Take lessons. Private tennis lessons can easily cost $60 an hour, says van der Sommen. A more affordable option is to take a clinic or class with no more than four students. Check out your local community college for tennis clinics and workshops.

Choose your court. Grass is the worst surface on which to learn tennis; clay is the best, according to van der Sommen. But if you're just starting out, look for an indoor court, he says. There will be no sun to blind you, no wind to skew your shots, and a less distracting background that enables you to better see the ball.

FAT BLASTER

Even if you can't find an opponent to play some days, you can still work on your game. Find a wall to hit balls against. Or rent a ball machine to send balls whizzing at you on the court.

Tennis Workouts

Beginner	**Intermediate**	**Experienced**
Enjoy noncompetitive play for at least ½ hour against someone of equal or greater ability than yourself.	Play competitively for 45 minutes to an hour.	Engage in an hour to 90 minutes of tournament-type play.

WALKING

Calories Burned

100 per mile

Body-Shaping Potential

Tones abdominals, hips, thighs, and buttocks

Here's what you can expect when you walk regularly.

▶ Your body will burn more calories and more fat all day long because you've revved up your metabolism.

▶ You'll help tone your abdominals, hips, thighs, and buttocks.

▶ You'll use all the major muscles—glutes, quads, hamstrings, back, biceps, and triceps.

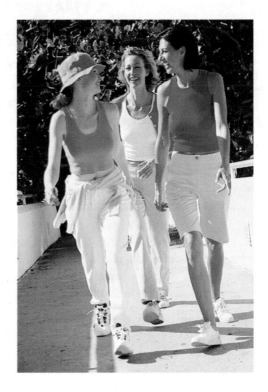

On Your Feet

Priority one for all walkers is good shoes. Here is what nationally known racewalker and instructor Bonnie Stein recommends that you look for when you shop for shoes.

Flexibility. The shoe should bend where your foot bends—at the ball of your foot, not in the middle of the shoe.

An ample toebox. When you walk, you bend and push off with your toes. There should be a thumb's width from the end of your longest toe to the front end of the shoe, says Stein. If the toebox isn't big enough, your toes will be tingling 20 minutes into your walk.

Light, thin materials. Look for shoes that are lightweight, with a thin heel and a flexible sole. Running and walking shoes with soles that are extremely thick and cushioned are not good for walking. Also stay away

from aerobics, tennis, and basketball shoes, Stein says. Cross-trainers are too stiff and inflexible for walking and don't offer the proper support.

Other Stuff You'll Need

If you venture outdoors on your walks, you'll want to be prepared for any conditions.

Water. Drink 2 cups (16 ounces) of water about 2 hours prior to your workout, then 5 to 10 ounces every 15 to 20 minutes during exercise. After you're done, drink 16 ounces for

Real Women
SHOW YOU HOW

Karen Whittled Her Weight by Walking

Barely 5 feet tall, 47-year-old Karen Primerano wore size 14 jeans. She had tried to lose weight by consuming diet foods and liquid diet drinks, but she always managed to regain any weight that she lost. After several years of unsuccessful dieting, she had finally had enough.

"One day," says Karen, "I said to my husband, 'That's it. I've spent my last nickel on anything diet.' So we went out and bought a treadmill.

"I was so out of shape that it took me months to work up to walking 20 minutes. In the beginning, I couldn't walk for even 5 minutes at a slow pace without being totally out of breath," she recalls. But she stuck with it.

Every week, she increased her treadmill time by 1 minute, until she was up to 20 minutes at a time. She used the treadmill every night during the week, and on weekends, she walked 2 to 3 miles around her neighborhood.

As the weeks went by, the pounds started easing off. Karen lost 40 pounds, and she was able to trade in her size 14 jeans for a slim size 6.

---

each pound of weight lost during the workout.

Sun protection. Wear sunscreen and a floppy, wide-brimmed hat or baseball cap, sunglasses with 100 percent ultraviolet protection, or a visor to shade your eyes and protect your face from sunburn. A visor is best for really hot weather because it doesn't hold the heat in.

Wet-weather gear. There's plenty of rain gear available to make wet-weather walking enjoyable. You can also find wet-weather activewear in mail-order catalogs such as Eddie Bauer and L. L. Bean.

Cold-weather gear. When it's cold outside, you want clothing made with a fabric that pulls the moisture away from your skin. Look for T-shirts, turtlenecks, and other attire made with CoolMax or other synthetic fibers designed for activewear. You can dress in layers, but don't wear cotton next to your skin, because it won't wick away the sweat. Cover your ears with a headband or a hat. Just be aware that even at a cool 35° or 40°F, a hat may make your head perspire, so a headband is a better choice. When the temperatures dip below freezing, however, wear a hat. When the weather is cool, you may want to wear gloves. When it gets really cold, switch to mittens. Stein likes polar fleece for headbands and mittens because it doesn't trap moisture.

Getting Started

With your walking shoes firmly on your feet, it is time to hit the road. Here are some pointers from Stein.

Take it slow. If you need to lose 50 or more pounds or you are relatively inactive, don't overdo it at first. Aim for a daily 20-minute walk at a pace that makes your breathing just a bit labored but doesn't leave you out of breath. "At the end of 20 minutes, you'll probably feel great, as though you could do more—but don't," says Stein. "In the first 2 to 3 weeks of walking, don't go more than 20 minutes per session."

Plan to walk every day. "Even on days when you don't feel like doing it, just get out and walk a few blocks," says Stein. You'd be surprised at how, once you get going, those few blocks can turn into a mile or more.

To maximize the body-shaping benefits of walking, follow these tips from Kate Larsen, a walking instructor and certified group fitness instructor in Minneapolis.

Take short, quick steps instead of long strides. You'll work your glute muscles (in your buttocks) as you log miles.

Practice using the heel-toe roll. Push off from your heel, roll through the outside of your foot, then push through your big toe. Think of your big toe as the Go button and push off with propulsion. Keep your other toes relaxed.

"Zip up" your abs. During your walk, imagine that you're zipping up a tight pair of jeans. Stand tall and pull your abdominal muscles up and in. This will also strengthen your lower-back muscles.

Pump your arms. Imagine that you're holding the rubber grips of ski poles in your hands. Stand straight, drop your shoulders, squeeze your shoulder blades behind you, and push your elbows back with each step. Keep your arm movements smooth and strong, moving past the outside of your hips.

Hold your head up. Look about 10 feet ahead of you. Imagine that you're wearing a baseball cap with the bill of the visor level to the horizon, so that you have to look up just enough to see the road. This keeps your neck aligned properly.

FAT BLASTER

Imagine squeezing and lifting your glutes up and back, as if you were holding a $50 bill between them. This will strengthen and tone your glute muscles. Developing the ability to maintain this deep contraction throughout your walk will take a while.

Walking Workouts

Beginner	Intermediate	Experienced
Walk for 20 minutes, 6 or 7 days a week for 2 weeks	Walk for 25 minutes, 6 or 7 days a week; increase walking time by 10 percent increments each week until you reach 40 minutes	Continue to increase walking time by 10 percent until you reach 45 to 60 minutes, 6 or 7 days a week. If you don't need to lose body fat, you can walk 20 to 30 minutes, 3 days a week to stay fit.

WATER AEROBICS

Calories Burned

200 to 250 per half-hour

Body-Shaping Potential

Tones abdominals, hips, thighs, buttocks, calves, arms, and more

Water workouts on a regular basis can bring you a steady stream of rewards.

▶ By engaging in an energetic water aerobics workout, you'll burn calories just as well as if you did an aerobic workout on land, without the added stress on your joints.

▶ The three-dimensional effects of water provide resistance in all directions, toning your muscles from head to toe. Water exercise creates a beautifully shaped and balanced body.

▶ You'll work your abdominal and back muscles, along with your legs, extra hard in the water to maintain erect body alignment and balance, resulting in strong, defined abdominals and legs.

On Your Feet

Water fitness shoes are soft, flexible shoes that are specifically designed for walking in water. They add comfort, provide a nonskid base, and help protect your feet. Water fitness sneakers, which provide more support than the shoes, are also a good choice. But if you like, you can do water aerobics in your bare feet.

Other Stuff You'll Need

Water aerobics requires minimal equipment. A bathing suit and a pool will do the trick. For

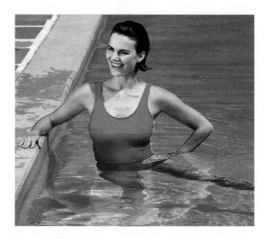

added efficiency and safety, you can opt for additional water aerobics equipment.

Water. A backyard pool or the one at the local Y are both perfect. The water should be approximately chest deep, and you should have enough space to move through a full range of motion without bumping into the side of the pool or the person next to you. Water temperature is important: The Aquatic Exercise Association says it should be 80° to 85°F for water fitness classes. As your body temperature rises from the vigorous parts of the routine, this temperature keeps you cool, explains Marti Boutin, a training specialist for the Aquatic Exercise Association, headquartered in Nokomis, Florida.

Swimsuit. Comfort is the key here. Wear a suit that you can move well in. If wearing a swimsuit makes you feel embarrassed because you're out of shape, just pull a T-shirt over your suit.

Resistance-training aids. Working out in the water tones your abs and helps to flatten your stomach. Adding other equipment, such as water dumbbells, Styrofoam noodles,

Real Women
SHOW YOU HOW

Linda Gets Hip to Water Aerobics

"**I** love to be active," says Linda Grable, a 50-plus office manager. Despite having been born with a dislocated hip that made her vulnerable to injury, she was a runner and worked out at a gym. Over the years, however, she developed arthritis in both hips. Her doctor recommended two hip replacements.

"Since the surgery, I haven't been able to do any exercises that may put stress on my hips," Linda says. "I can no longer run, use the step machine, or take aerobics classes. I had to explore different activities.

"One day, I got a flyer for a water aerobics class in the mail," Linda recalls. "I read the class description and thought about it for a few days. Then I decided, 'Hey, I'm going to do this!'" And she's thrilled that she did.

"Water aerobics finally allows me to do the things I used to be able to do on land," she says. "I felt so limited after surgery. Now, for the first time, I was able to do jogging and jumping jacks, lunges and kicks. I am so tickled!"

The 1-hour class is "a really, really good workout," Linda says. "It's almost constant movement, so I know I'm giving my heart a good workout." The class also incorporates resistance training for more-focused muscle toning.

and webbed gloves, helps tone other muscles groups—notably your thighs, buttocks, and arms—while increasing the intensity of your workout, Boutin says.

Flotation belt. For deep-water workouts (where your feet don't touch the bottom), a flotation belt is essential for safety, and it also provides good back support.

FAT BLASTER

Don't just do water walking and leave it at that. There's a huge range of things you can do in the water, from lap swimming to water yoga. By experimenting with new things, you sustain your interest.

Water Aerobics Workouts

Beginner	Intermediate	Experienced
Target heart rate 60 to 65 percent of maximum, 2 to 3 days a week.	Target heart rate 65 to 75 percent of maximum, 3 to 4 days a week.	Target heart rate 75 to 90 percent of maximum, 4 to 6 days a week.

YARD WORK

Calories Burned
Per 10 minutes: raking, 37; hedging, 52; mowing, 76

Body-Shaping Potential
Tones arms, shoulders, chest, back, buttocks, abdomen, and legs

The walking, bending, heaving, and hoeing of yard work engages almost all of your torso, leg, and arm muscles, says Barbara Ainsworth, Ph.D., associate professor of exercise science and director of the Prevention Research Center at the University of South Carolina in Columbia.

▶ You'll get a challenging, calorie-burning aerobic workout from mowing, raking, and other rigorous, rhythmic tasks.

▶ You'll work your back, chest, abdomen, buttocks, legs, arms, and shoulders by pushing a lawn mower or pulling a rake or hoe. Trimming bushes and trees gives your arms and back an even greater workout.

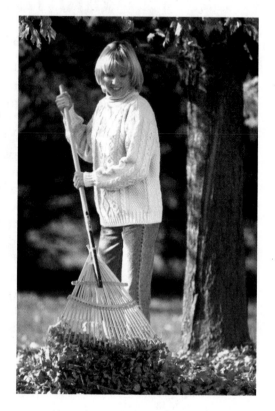

On Your Feet

Any activity that involves working with sharp tools on uneven terrain calls for protective footwear. Don't even think of tackling chores in a pair of flimsy loafers or canvas sneakers. Instead, lace up the sturdiest shoes you own—ones with hard soles and sturdy uppers. If you must, press your walking shoes or hiking boots into service for yard chores.

Other Stuff You'll Need

If you have a yard, you probably have at least a rake or two on hand, some kind of grass mower, and hand tools of some kind. Using the proper tools in the correct way can go a long way toward maximizing your yard "workout."

The right tools. Manual tools that you have to push or pull with your own strength will build strong legs while you firm your abdomen and buttocks. A push lawn mower instead of a riding mower or an old-fashioned rake instead of a motorized leaf-blower will help give you the workout you're looking for.

When buying tools like clippers or edgers, choose manual versions. Pay particular attention to your ergonomic comfort: Look for comfortable handles and angles that require effort yet don't put undue strain on your back or other parts of your body. If possible, opt for a manual mower or a self-propelled push mower.

The right clothes. What you wear can make all the difference between a good experience and a not-so-good one, even in your own backyard. In warmer weather, wear loose-fitting lightweight clothes that will breathe when you perspire. In cooler weather, dress in layers that you can easily take off or put back on as necessary.

Sun sense. Always wear a hat and sunscreen to protect against ultraviolet rays.

Getting Started

The grass is growing, and those dandelions are taking over the lawn. There's lots to be done and no time like the present. Here are some suggestions to help you tackle your yard.

Do a little at a time. If until now you've been paying the kid down the block to maintain your 2-acre spread, don't hand him a pink slip quite yet. Start out by taking over only

Real Women SHOW YOU HOW

Suzanne Trimmed Her Waist by Trimming Her Trees

When Suzanne DeJohn, 38, moved from Boston to rural Vermont 10 years ago, she couldn't wait to get outside and begin working in her new yard.

"I love being out in the fresh air, listening to the trees rustle," she says.

So fond is Suzanne of the outdoors that she took a job as a landscaper. For 5 years, she dug vegetable and flower beds, mowed lawns, raked leaves, and hauled dirt, mulch, and rocks. At the same time, she took to tending a garden of her own. It's hard work, she says, but it's fun. What's more, it's the best physical fitness regimen she has ever engaged in.

"Yard work is a great form of exercise," she says. "I feel my fitness level increase each year, and friends have even commented on my strong muscles and good health." Though no longer a landscaper, you can still find her out in her 3-acre yard every weekend and often on weekdays after work.

"I'd much rather work in the yard and garden than go to a gym. The fresh air is wonderful, and I find a certain peace of mind outdoors. When I'm finished, I have a sense of accomplishment. I have something to show for all my work, whether it's a new perennial bed or a big pile of leaves."

small portions of yard work and counting them as big accomplishments.

Warm up. Ease into light activity first, Dr. Ainsworth advises. "Don't immediately take the mower out and pull the crank on the engine. That's a huge strain on your back." Instead, do a few minutes of raking or some other activity that makes you gently move and stretch your whole body.

Vary your activities. Don't lean over the rake all weekend. In fact, don't engage in any single yard work activity for hours on end, says Dr. Ainsworth, or you'll risk stressing particular muscle groups and end up aching. Instead, break big tasks into smaller chunks of about 10 minutes each.

Get close to your tools. Tools such as trimmers and hedgers can be heavy, awkward, and dangerous. "These tools put a strain on your hand, arm, and back as they work to support the weight of the implement," Dr. Ainsworth explains. To reduce the strain, pull the tool in closer toward your body as you work with it.

Watch your back. The frequent bending involved in yard work can really put pressure on your back. Practice proper bending and lifting techniques, suggests Dr. Ainsworth. Instead of bending at the waist, squat down with your legs, and lift back up with your legs instead of your back.

Switch sides. Give the muscles on both sides of your body a good workout. "Do your raking from the left, then switch to the right, and keep alternating periodically," suggests Dr. Ainsworth. "Otherwise, you'll end up out of balance, with one side of your body noticeably stronger than the other. There's also more risk of muscle strain if you stick to one side."

Drink a lot of water. Don't just water the grass. Water yourself frequently with a swig from a water bottle. If you don't, you'll risk dehydration, which can cause fatigue and muscle cramps.

FAT BLASTER

As you grow stronger, you can come up with new ways to make yard work even more of a workout, suggests Richard Cotton, chief exercise physiologist for the American Council on Exercise in San Diego. "Try walking a little faster behind your mower," he suggests. "Or switch from a power saw to a manual pruner for a great forearm and hand workout."

Yard Work Workouts

Beginner	Intermediate	Experienced
Watering and seeding a lawn for 10 minutes, two or three times a week	Mowing with a self-propelled push mower, raking, or trimming shrubs or trees for 30 minutes at a time, three times a week	Digging, spreading fertilizer, or mowing with a manual mower or doing other chores for 35 to 45 minutes, four or five times a week

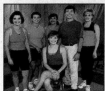
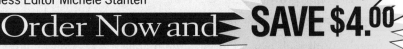

Chapter 6

Flatten Your Abs and Slenderize Your Waist

See results in as little as 4 weeks!

I f you are not happy with your belly and waist, know that you are not alone. In a survey of more than 500 women, two-thirds of the women—a whopping 67 percent—cited their bellies as trouble zones. Among the same women, 40 percent cited their waists as problem areas.

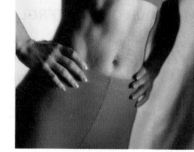

Your abdominal muscles confine your internal organs like a snug girdle. But pregnancy can present a challenge to these muscles.

As a baby grows within the womb, the surrounding abdominal muscles—especially the lower abs—stretch . . . and stretch . . . and stretch. With each passing month, the muscle fibers lose strength and elasticity. If you have a second or third baby, the process repeats itself. If you have a cesarean delivery, in which the muscles are surgically separated, the muscles become weaker still, losing their ability to expand and contract. When you add them up, these changes mean that your muscles lose their tone. The result is a postpregnancy belly bulge.

Even if you've never been pregnant, your tummy can protrude, especially when you approach menopause. Researchers aren't sure why, but the drop in female sex hormones that heralds menopause prompts fat to accumulate over your abs. If you're overweight all over, your abs may be temporarily obscured by an extra layer of fat.

With the Banish Your Belly, Butt, and Thighs program, you can tighten and tone those ab muscles, restoring (or even improving) your figure.

4 Weeks to a Flatter Belly

Anything that you can do to tighten your abdominal muscles will help hold in your stomach and other organs. Your abs consist of four muscles, all of which shape your torso.

▶ The rectus abdominus (upper and lower), a vertical muscle that runs from your rib cage to your pubic bone

▶ The transverse abdominus, the deepest ab, which runs horizontally across your torso

▶ The external oblique, a broad, thin muscle that runs diagonally from your ribs to your hip

▶ The internal oblique muscle, which runs along the front and sides of your torso

The upper and lower abs and the obliques are "helper" muscles: You can press them into service as needed. If you're lying on your back on the beach and you reach forward to apply sunscreen to your knees, you're working your upper abs. If you're lying on the floor watching TV and you raise your legs, you're working your lower abs. If you're standing at the office photocopier and you bend to

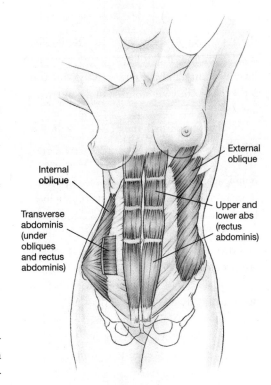

Internal oblique

External oblique

Transverse abdominis (under obliques and rectus abdominis)

Upper and lower abs (rectus abdominis)

To slim your waist and flatten your stomach, you need to work the upper and lower abs and the oblique muscles in the abdominal area. That's exactly what our program does.

the right or left, you're working your obliques.

The trouble is, we don't routinely tax our abdominal muscles very much during the course of a day. But if we worked them harder, or more often, or both, they would tighten up and get stronger, and our tummies wouldn't protrude.

To slim your waist and tummy distended by pregnancy, overweight, or hormonal changes, you need a program of exercises that deliberately work the abs—especially the upper and lower abs and the obliques—as well as a weight-loss regimen to lose excess fat. Working the abs as you go about your daily duties helps, too. Combine the following program with healthy eating and aerobic activity, and you'll see a change in your stomach and waist within a month.

"The abdominal muscles are wonderful muscle groups to work on because they respond very quickly to exercise," says Marjorie Albohm, an exercise physiologist, certified athletic trainer, and director of sports medicine at Kendrick Memorial Hospital in Mooresville, Indiana. "Compared to your buttocks, thighs, or other muscle groups, the abs get stronger pretty quickly."

The workouts that follow produce results because they use the principle of overload. That is, the only way to tone and strengthen a muscle is to boost the effort by increasing either duration (by doing more repetitions) or intensity (by doing the same number of reps but adding weights to make the exercise harder). If you're new to exercise, start at the beginner level. If you are able to complete the designated program with relative ease for three consecutive workout sessions, then it's time to progress to the next level.

"You'll feel results in about 2 weeks," says Albohm. "By 4 weeks, you should see some tightening or slight changes in contour. And by 6 weeks, you'll look and feel toned."

Women who have had children are eager to regain their prepregnancy shapes, Albohm notes, but this may take more effort. "Because the abs stretch to support the size of a fetus, it's hard for your tummy to return to its prepregnancy level. By working your abs, though, you can tighten the muscles that have been stretched and regain muscle tone."

Real Women
SHOW YOU HOW

She Slowed It Down

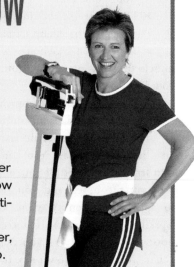

Eight months after the birth of her second child, Janine Slaughter, 38, wanted her prebaby body back, but nothing seemed to work, including the 100 crunches she did each day. Janine's secret to trimming 2 inches off her waist? Instead of doing 100 crunches quickly, she slowed down to make her muscles do the work. "Now that I've learned to slow down and really concentrate on holding each repetition, I'm doing fewer exercises, but my stomach is flatter and firmer!" she says. Now 9 pounds trimmer, Janine has a tighter tummy and a bigger smile, too.

Maximum Results with Minimum Effort

To make sure that you get the results you're after, Albohm suggests doing these torso-shaping workouts in front of a mirror so you can check your position. "If you've never exercised before, you may have no idea what position your head, neck, shoulders, and back are in, or how far off the floor you are," she explains.

Here are some other workout tips from Albohm for getting the fastest results with the least effort.

Work all the abs. If you're trying to regain muscle tone after pregnancy, you will probably want to focus more on the lower abs. But don't neglect the others. As a rule, you should work the upper and lower abs and the obliques equally.

Flex those knees. If you don't, you're likely to use your hip muscles, not your abs, which will defeat the purpose of the exercise. As you advance, you may be doing straight-leg raises.

Flatten your back. You should flatten your back against the floor to protect your lower-back muscles against strain. You'll probably want to use an exercise mat, but a carpeted floor or a large folded towel may work just as well.

Start easy. Three to 10 repetitions is the maximum for beginners.

Use slow, controlled movements. Use slow, steady movements and hold each position for a count of two, suggests Albohm. If you experience pain or discomfort when performing an exercise, stop and substitute another version, she advises. If pain persists, see your physician.

Be consistent. "Next to performing the exercises correctly, exercising regularly is key," says Albohm. The beginner, intermediate, and experienced workouts outlined in "How Much, How Often?" should be done three or four times a week.

Combine ab work with diet and aerobics. "You can't say, 'I want to take 3 inches off my waist,' do 500 ab exercises and nothing else, and expect it to work—it won't," says Albohm. If you ignore aerobic exercise—and a sensible diet—your belly will show it.

Combining aerobics with ab workouts helps in two ways: The combination burns calories, which helps get rid of excess weight all over, including the abdomen, and it gives your abs a little boost.

"The fact that you're supporting your body as you move forces the muscles to contract," explains Albohm. "If you deliberately contract your abs during aerobic exercise, you'll benefit even more."

Be patient. "Don't expect results overnight. If you're a beginner, start at the beginner level. When working at one level becomes easy and effortless, move on to the next," says Albohm.

How Much, How Often?

Beginner: 1 set of 3 to 10 reps, 3 days per week
Intermediate: 2 sets of 10 reps, 3 days per week
Experienced: 3 or 4 sets of 10 reps, 3 or 4 days per week

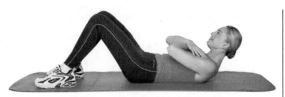

Mini-crunch: Lie on your back with your knees bent and your arms crossed in front of your chest. Slowly lift your head and shoulders off the floor together (do not bend your neck). Don't lift beyond your shoulder blades coming off the floor. Hold and then lower.

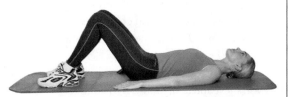

Pelvic tuck: Lie on your back with your knees bent. Tightening your abs, tilt your pelvis so that your back is pressed to the floor. Hold for a few seconds and then release. Once you've mastered this on the floor, learn to do it standing. This is the position that your pelvis should be in to stabilize your back when doing standing exercises.

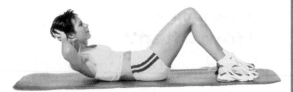

Abdominal crunch: Lie on the floor with your knees bent and feet flat on the floor. Place your hands loosely behind your head. Slowly curl your shoulders about 30 degrees off the floor. Hold, then slowly lower.

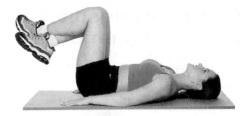

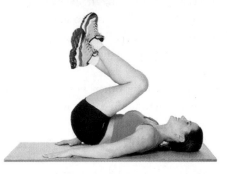

Reverse curl: Bend your hips and knees so that your legs are over your midsection and relaxed. Slowly contract your abdominal muscles, lifting your hips 2 to 4 inches off the floor. Slowly lower.

Back Pain? Avoid These Exercises

If you have any type of back pain, these exercises will do more to hurt your already aching back than help. Avoid them.

- Full situps
- Straight-leg situps
- Deadlifts and good mornings
- Overhead presses
- Unsupported forward flexions
- Trunk twists
- Hyperextensions

Real Women
SHOW YOU HOW

She Takes Exercise Breaks

After 15 years of being unhappy with her weight, Rita Blanks, 55, wanted her waistline back, but she needed a program that fit into a life jam-packed with work and family. After adopting a regimen of aerobics and weight training, Rita also traded coffee breaks for stretching breaks and began adding exercise to her life wherever she could. "I do isometric exercises while sitting at my desk—contracting and releasing certain muscles. And I do calf raises while standing at the copier," she says. "You'd be surprised how much exercise you can squeeze into a day!" Now 18 pounds lighter, Rita has her waistline back for good.

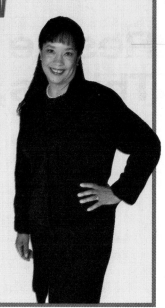

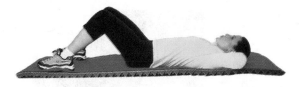

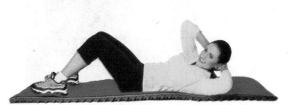

Diagonal curl-up: Slowly lift your head and shoulders off the floor, twist to the left, and bring your right shoulder toward your left knee. Slowly lower. Repeat, alternating sides.

FAT BLASTER

Waiting in line? Sitting at your desk? Use this time to work your abs. While standing or sitting, contract your upper abdominals by inhaling sharply and holding in the muscles. Breathing normally, hold for 6 to 8 seconds, then release.

Chapter 7

Resize Your Hips, Thighs, and Buttocks

See results in 30 days!

Any physiology teacher will tell you that, by nature's design, women are programmed to have wider lower bodies than men. We need wider pelvic bones for childbearing and to support a growing fetus—and sturdy thighs and generous backsides to support *us* while we carry the growing fetus for 9 months. Add a genetically programmed layer of fat, and you have your mom's hips, thighs, and buttocks.

"Most women, even if they're not overly pear-shaped, will gain weight in their hips and thighs before they gain it anywhere else," points out Marjorie Albohm, an exercise physiologist, certified athletic trainer, and director of sports medicine at Kendrick Memorial Hospital in Mooresville, Indiana. "Men accumulate fat in the abdominal area, and women accumulate fat in the hip and thigh area—that's a fact. All you have to do is look at lots of men and women the next time you are in a crowd or go to the mall. That's how fat is distributed between the genders."

Heavier hips, thighs, and buttocks are more a factor of gender than age. "Whether they're 20 or 40, women still have 10 to 15 percent more body fat than men, even if they work out," says Albohm.

While that might make sense, it doesn't make us happy. In a survey of 500 women conducted for this publication, nearly half said they wished they had slimmer thighs, and more than 40 percent said they were dissatisfied with their hips. A fair number—25 percent—said they regarded their backsides as a trouble zone.

It's not that these women want to look like guys, with narrow hips, a flat butt, and wide shoulders. But we would like to have shapelier

lower bodies and not let genetics take over completely. And that's where our program comes in.

See the Difference in Just 1 Month

To tone and trim your hips, thighs, and buttocks, you need a total-body workout with special emphasis on the muscle groups that you want to tone, says Albohm, who designs workout programs specifically for women who want to do something about the weight they carry on their hips and thighs. "Your goal is to

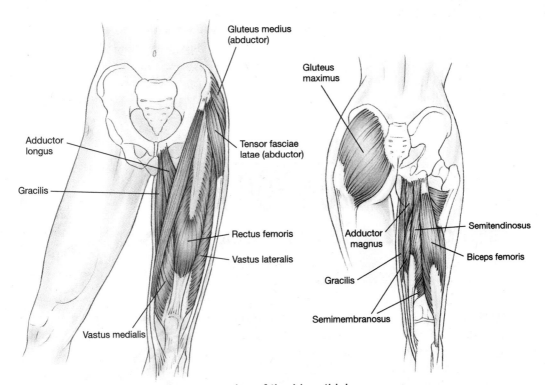

The primary muscles of the hips, thighs, and buttocks dictate their shape (and size). The more you tone these muscles, the less prominent they appear.

change the circumference of this area." Combined with some kind of consistent aerobic exercise—and eating habits that subtract pounds—the workouts that follow can help you reach your goal, she says. If you're just starting to exercise, start at the beginner level (see "How Much, How Often?"). If you are able to complete a designated program with relative ease for three consecutive workout sessions, then it's time to proceed to the next level.

You can expect to see some change in as little as 30 days, says Albohm.

As with any exercise, there's a right and a wrong way to go about working your hips, thighs, and buttocks.

Easy does it—at first. Start with the beginner program until you get used to the movements, says Albohm. If you decide to add ankle weights to work your inner and outer thigh muscles, start with light weights and only a few reps. Don't exceed 5 pounds—you completely change the leverage on your joints.

Do the exercise correctly to avoid injury. If you arch your back while you're doing the hip extension, for example, you could strain your back. And don't cheat—complete the full range of motion.

Make yourself comfortable. For some of the exercises that are done on the floor, you'll probably want to use an exercise mat. If you don't have a mat, a carpeted floor or large, folded towel may work just as well. But if you experience pain or discomfort when performing an exercise, stop and substitute another version, advises Albohm. If pain persists, see your physician.

Keep your movements tight and controlled. Don't swing your way through the exercise or let your muscles go slack.

Work your whole body. "Despite what you may have heard, if it's strenuous enough—if you walk like you really mean it, for example—aerobic exercise can tone your muscles to some degree," says Albohm. "I do aero-

Real Women
SHOW YOU HOW

She Got Results in 1 Week

After only a few 5-minute sessions doing the opposite arm and leg lift, Danielle Kost's lower back got stronger. She used to hunch over her keyboard, but now she sits up straight all day—comfortably. She says it's as if there's a brace on her back, giving her spine extra support and keeping her posture correct—without her having to think about it.

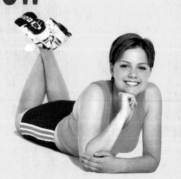

bics primarily for the cardiovascular effects, for example. But 20 to 30 percent of my effort carries over to strengthen and tone my muscles."

Step right up. Step aerobics is better for the hips, thighs, and buttocks than regular aerobics, because it involves the quads, adductors, abductors, and gluteals, says Albohm. Stairclimbing machines are good for the quads, hamstrings, and gluteals—you work up and down in a straight line.

If you use a stairclimber, program the machine to vary the resistance and height to give your muscles a thorough workout, recommends Albohm. (The same advice applies if you use an elliptical trainer or recumbent bike.)

Measure your progress. It's a good idea to measure your hips, thighs, and buttocks every month, not every week, says Albohm. "Just be sure to measure at the same spot, in the same way, every time." And don't worry that your hips, thighs, and buttocks will get bigger when you follow this program. "Weight training will make muscles bigger only if it's done for that reason. These exercises don't do that."

Be consistent. "To get the fastest results in the shortest period of time, do the exercises exactly as shown and make them part of your life," says Albohm.

How Much, How Often?

Beginner: 1 set of 3 to 10 reps, 3 days per week
Intermediate: 2 sets of 10 reps, 3 days per week
Experienced: 3 sets of 10 reps, 3 days per week

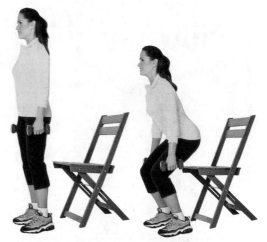

Squat: Bending at the knees and hips, lower yourself as though you're sitting down. Keep your back straight, and make sure you can always see your toes. Stop just shy of touching the chair, then stand back up.

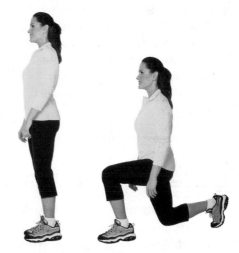

Lunge: Standing with your feet together, step back 2 to 3 feet with your right foot. Bending your left knee, slowly lower yourself. Keep your left knee directly over your ankle. Before your right knee touches the floor, push off with your right foot, and return to the starting position. Repeat with your left leg.

Real Women
SHOW YOU HOW

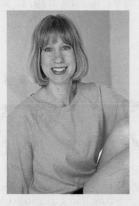

No More Jiggle!

Lauri Centolanza felt her inner thighs jiggle the first time she did an inner thigh lift. But after just 3 weeks, she noticed less jiggle. "This move is so easy to do that I've added it—along with outer thigh raises—to my after-run routine. My thighs look toned!" she says.

FAT BLASTER

Work your butt and legs by taking the stairs. If you have stairs at work, climb one flight for 3 weeks. Then increase the number of flights by one every 3 weeks. Or walk up and down the stairs in your home three to five extra times each day.

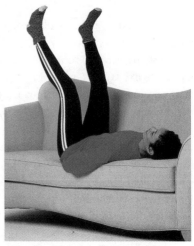

Scissors: Lie on your back on a couch (you may need to angle yourself for more room) with your hands (palms down) under your butt and your legs straight up in the air. Keeping your knees slightly bent and your feet flexed, slowly spread your legs as far apart as comfortable. Hold, then slowly bring your legs together, resisting as you press them in.

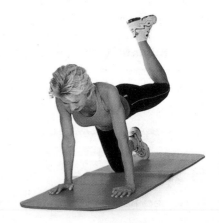

Hip extension: Get down on all fours, with your back flat. Keeping your knees bent and squeezing your butt, lift your left leg until it's in line with your spine. Slowly lower. Complete one set before switching sides and repeating with your right leg.

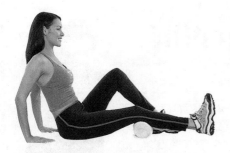 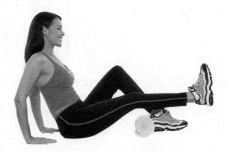

Straight leg lift: Sitting on the floor, lean back slightly, and place your hands a few inches behind your butt. Keep a slight bend in your elbows. Extend your legs straight in front of you. Bend your left knee so that your left foot is on the floor next to your right leg, just above the ankle. Place a rolled towel under your right knee to help maintain a slight bend in your knee as you perform the move.

Without bending your leg any farther, slowly lift your right leg as high as possible. This may be as little as 4 to 6 inches in the beginning and as much as 12 to 16 inches when you become stronger and more flexible. Keep your toes pointing up. Hold, then slowly lower. Complete one set before switching sides and repeating with your other leg.

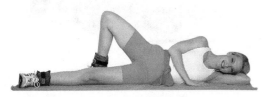 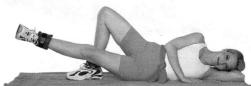

Inner thigh lift: Wearing ankle weights, lie on an exercise mat on your left side, with your left leg straight. Bend your right leg so the knee is pointing toward the ceiling and your right foot is flat on the floor just behind your left knee. You can lean back slightly so that you're lying halfway on your left buttock. Rest your head on your bent left arm, and lightly place your right hand on the floor in front of you for balance.

Looking straight ahead and keeping your shoulders and hips aligned, slowly lift your left leg to about shoulder height. Keep your abdominals tight and your foot flexed. Hold, then slowly lower. Repeat for one set before switching sides and repeating with your right leg.

Real Women
SHOW YOU HOW

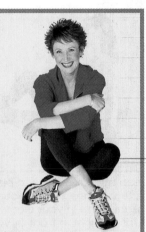

Hills? No Problem

Ellen Mazo thought she had strong legs—until she changed her running route. While trying to go up a winding, steep hill, she couldn't do it without stopping. But after 2 weeks of doing straight leg lifts, she can get up that slope, and her legs aren't tired after a long run. "I can tackle hills easily," she says. "And I also like the definition in my thighs!"

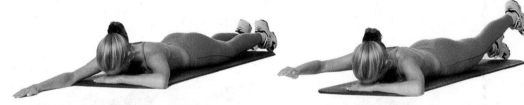

Opposite arm and leg lift: Lie face-down on the floor. Extend your right arm straight out in front of your head with your palm facing the floor. Use your left arm to support your forehead. The tip of your nose should nearly touch the floor, so that your neck and spine form a straight line.

At the same time, slowly lift your right arm, head, chest, and left leg off the floor. Your arm and leg should be raised approximately 4 to 5 inches, while your chest is raised only 2 to 3 inches. Tuck your chin slightly to keep your head, neck, and back in line. Hold for a second, then slowly lower. Repeat until you have done the desired number of reps with your right arm and left leg, then do the same number with your left arm and right leg.

NEW Video! from **_PREVENTION_**.

Burn Fat Faster!

Get Real Results in Just 2 Weeks!

Get a toned and trim body faster than you ever thought possible…with *Prevention* magazine's strength training video! It's the all-new workout for *real* women that shows you exactly how to do each move for fast results—with no injuries!

PLUS…

► **BURN MORE CALORIES**
► **BUILD STRONG BONES**
► **LOWER YOUR CHOLESTEROL**

Real Women Show You How

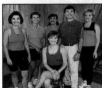

"I lost 11 pounds and 5 inches off my waist."
Rita Blanks, 54, mother of four, and grandmother of six

⁂ *Expert Advice from*
► Dr. Wayne L. Westcott, PhD
► *Prevention*'s Fitness Editor Michele Stanten

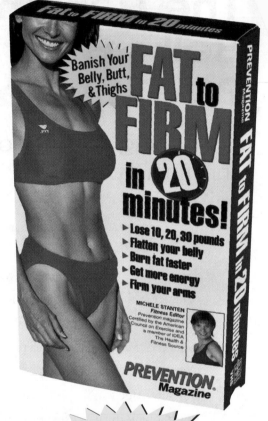

Banish Your Belly, Butt, & Thighs **FAT to FIRM in 20 minutes!**
► Lose 10, 20, 30 pounds
► Flatten your belly
► Burn fat faster
► Get more energy
► Firm your arms

MICHELE STANTEN
Fitness Editor
Prevention magazine
Certified by the American Council on Exercise and a member of IDEA, The Health & Fitness Source

PREVENTION Magazine®

Order Now and ⇒ SAVE $4.⁰⁰

(SUGGESTED RETAIL PRICE OF $19.95)   YOU PAY <u>ONLY</u> $15.95 + $1 HANDLING CHARGE

PZ 0201

Ordered by (please print)

Name _____

Address _____

City _____ State/Prov. _____ Zip/Postal Code _____

Daytime Phone (   )

Please enclose your <u>personal check</u> or <u>money order</u> payable to *Prevention* Magazine. Sorry, no credit card orders accepted. Send this form (or a copy) and your payment to **Shop Prevention!**, P.O. Box 7029, Emmaus, PA 18098. *Please allow 6 to 8 weeks for delivery. Thank you!*

Banish Your Belly, Butt, and Thighs 30-Day Planner

Everything you need to lose weight and firm up.

You are about to embark on a 30-day adventure.

Not only will you be thinner at the end of your journey, but you'll have also shed old bad habits and replaced them with new healthy ones. You will be a new person in body, that's for sure. But you'll also be brimming with a new spirit—a spirit of accomplishment, of confidence, of knowing that you can lose weight and keep it off. The next 30 days will witness a transformation of both your body and mental outlook.

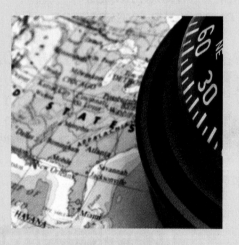

You'll have as your travel guide the Banish Your Belly, Butt, and Thighs 30-Day Planner. This day-to-day road map will provide information, inspiration, and direction for becoming the new and improved you. On the following pages, you'll find a handy checklist to track each day's diet and exercise accomplishments. We've packed the planner with nearly 90 tips on working out, eating right, and staying motivated. This planner will serve not only as a daily reminder of your weight-loss and toning goals but also as a record of your day-to-day triumphs and long-term progress.

This planner makes weight loss simple, uncomplicated, safe, and long lasting at the rate of a pound or two a week. (That's 10 to 20 pounds in just 10 weeks.)

One pound represents 3,500 calories. So to lose that 1 pound a week, you need to eliminate 3,500 calories—about 500 a day. The best way to cut out 500 calories is through a combination of diet and exercise. For example, stop drinking your afternoon soda. That's 200 calories right there. Then take a 3-mile walk or a 30-minute jog, and you've eliminated another 300. With just those two changes, you've cut out that 500 calories a day you need to lose weight.

It's that simple, and even easier with your planner companion. The next 30 pages will keep you on course as you lose the weight; get stronger; banish your belly, butt, and thighs; lower your cholesterol; and become a healthier, happier you. Enjoy the trip!

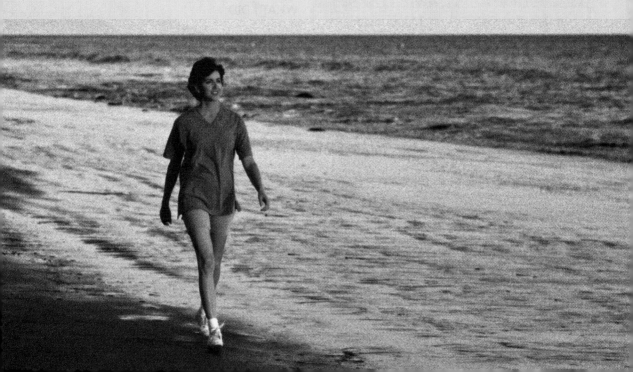

Date:

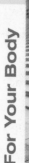 **For Your Body**

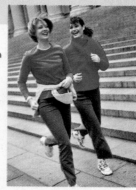

FOR YOUR MIND

Motivate with music. Mood affects eating and music affects mood. The upshot? If you're angry and heading for the cookie jar, stop at the stereo first. Try Pachelbel's Canon in D to soothe stress, anxiety, and a desire to eat. If you're feeling too weary to work out, put on "Johnny B. Goode" by Chuck Berry. By the second verse, you'll have trouble staying in your seat.

Take a moment to write down your accomplishments. Every day has one, and you'll feel better if you write them down daily, especially since it takes time to see the pounds come off. Today's could be as simple as "I started my weight-loss program!"

Set the bar low. What's the best way to stick with your commitment to exercise? Set the right goals! And in this case, think small. Wanting to run a marathon is a great goal, but it may take weeks or months to achieve. That's too long before you feel successful. So set lots of little goals, too, like "I want to run around the block without needing CPR" or "I want to do something physical every day."

Checklist

DAILY SERVINGS

5 vegetables ☐☐☐☐☐

4 fruits ☐☐☐☐

3–6 whole grains ☐☐☐☐☐☐

2–3 high-calcium foods ☐☐☐

8 glasses of water ☐☐☐☐ ☐☐☐☐

1 cup of tea ☐

DAILY SUPPLEMENT NEEDS

Multivitamin/mineral ☐
100% DV for most nutrients

Vitamin C: 100–500 mg ☐

Vitamin E: 100–400 IU ☐

Calcium: 500 mg ☐

WEEKLY SERVINGS

5+ beans ☐☐☐☐☐

5 nuts ☐☐☐☐☐

2 fish ☐☐

WHAT I DID:

☐ Abs and Waist Workout (pp. 134–39)

☐ Hips, Thighs, and Buttocks Workout (pp. 140–46)

☐ Aerobic Workout (pp. 64–132)

HOW I FELT: (what worked, what didn't)

_____
_____
_____
_____
_____
_____

WHAT I ATE:

_____
_____
_____
_____
_____

I'M PROUD OF:

_____
_____
_____
_____
_____

DAY 2

Date:

FOR THE RECORD

Focus on food. Since you're just starting out, record everything you eat. You can do it in a journal, on an index card or scrap of paper, or on this page. You may be surprised about which nutritional areas you come up short in . . . and how much "worthless" food you actually eat. Use the results to identify problem areas in your eating habits.

Tastebud trickery: Sucking on a menthol/eucalyptus cough drop can stop cravings instantly.

For Your Plate

Prime the pantry. Stock your kitchen with healthy foods—now! Your pantry should include such healthful staples as canned beans, whole wheat pasta and couscous, brown rice, white onions, canned tomatoes, low-sodium and low-fat stock or broth, plenty of dried spices, balsamic vinegar, olive or canola oil, and nonfat cooking spray.

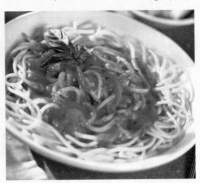

Checklist

DAILY SERVINGS

5 vegetables ☐☐☐☐☐

4 fruits ☐☐☐☐

3–6 whole ☐☐☐☐☐☐
grains

2–3 high-calcium ☐☐☐
foods

8 glasses ☐☐☐☐
of water ☐☐☐☐

1 cup of tea ☐

DAILY SUPPLEMENT NEEDS

Multivitamin/mineral ☐
100% DV for most nutrients

Vitamin C: 100–500 mg ☐

Vitamin E: 100–400 IU ☐

Calcium: 500 mg ☐

WEEKLY SERVINGS

5+ beans ☐☐☐☐☐

5 nuts ☐☐☐☐☐

2 fish ☐☐

WHAT I DID:

☐ Abs and Waist Workout (pp. 134–39)

☐ Hips, Thighs, and Buttocks Workout (pp. 140–46)

☐ Aerobic Workout (pp. 64–132)

HOW I FELT: (what worked, what didn't)

_____
_____
_____
_____
_____
_____
_____

WHAT I ATE:

_____
_____
_____
_____

I'M PROUD OF:

_____
_____
_____
_____

Date:

 FOR YOUR MIND

Accentuate the positive. Don't beat yourself up, no matter how your diet and exercise plans go awry on any given day. If you did your whole workout yesterday but can only manage half of it today, you haven't failed—you've been active 2 days in a row, and that's great!

Mirror, mirror . . . Chowing down in front of your reflection brings you face-to-face with your harshest critic: yourself. When you confront your mirror image, you're reminded of your goals, and you may think twice about what you eat.

For Your Body

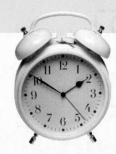

Alarm yourself. If you're afraid you won't get out of bed to do your morning workout, here's a fail-safe plan: Set three alarm clocks—the kind that keep beeping until you turn them off. Put one just outside the bedroom door so that you have to get out of bed to turn it off. Place another in the hallway and the third in the kitchen. By the time you turn them all off, you'll be awake . . . and less likely to throw in the towel.

Checklist

DAILY SERVINGS

5 vegetables ☐☐☐☐☐

4 fruits ☐☐☐☐

3–6 whole grains ☐☐☐☐☐

2–3 high-calcium foods ☐☐☐

8 glasses of water ☐☐☐☐ ☐☐☐☐

1 cup of tea ☐

DAILY SUPPLEMENT NEEDS

Multivitamin/mineral ☐
100% DV for most nutrients

Vitamin C: 100–500 mg ☐

Vitamin E: 100–400 IU ☐

Calcium: 500 mg ☐

WEEKLY SERVINGS

5+ beans ☐☐☐☐☐

5 nuts ☐☐☐☐☐

2 fish ☐☐

WHAT I DID:

☐ Abs and Waist Workout (pp. 134–39)

☐ Hips, Thighs, and Buttocks Workout (pp. 140–46)

☐ Aerobic Workout (pp. 64–132)

HOW I FELT: (what worked, what didn't)

_____
_____
_____
_____
_____
_____

WHAT I ATE:

_____
_____
_____
_____
_____

I'M PROUD OF:

_____
_____
_____
_____
_____

DAY 4

Date:

FOR THE RECORD

Count 'em up.

You may be shocked to find out exactly how many calories and grams of fat you consume in a day—or you may be pleasantly surprised. Either way, use a nutrition guide to tally up your totals from yesterday's food list.

The under story: Don't wear cotton panties and bras under tops and shorts made from wicking fabrics like CoolMax and Dri-FIT. The best wicking fabrics won't do much if they're on top of cotton, which stays wet.

For Your Plate

Make perfect low-fat pizza.
If you've ever tried to melt low-fat mozzarella on pizza, you may have wound up with something more akin to rubber than cheese. Well, here's a trick to keep your cheese cheesy: Spritz the cheese with a 3-second mist of cooking spray before heating. This little bit of extra fat on the surface of low-fat or fat-free cheese makes the cheese creamy when it melts, without adding calories.

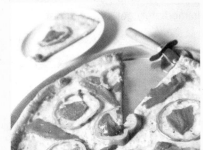

Checklist

DAILY SERVINGS

5 vegetables	☐☐☐☐☐
4 fruits	☐☐☐☐
3–6 whole grains	☐☐☐☐☐☐
2–3 high-calcium foods	☐☐☐
8 glasses of water	☐☐☐☐ ☐☐☐☐
1 cup of tea	☐

DAILY SUPPLEMENT NEEDS

Multivitamin/mineral ☐
100% DV for most nutrients
Vitamin C: 100–500 mg ☐
Vitamin E: 100–400 IU ☐
Calcium: 500 mg ☐

WEEKLY SERVINGS

5+ beans	☐☐☐☐☐
5 nuts	☐☐☐☐☐
2 fish	☐☐

WHAT I ATE:

_____
_____
_____
_____
_____
_____

WHAT I DID:

☐ Abs and Waist Workout (pp. 134–39)
☐ Hips, Thighs, and Buttocks Workout (pp. 140–46)
☐ Aerobic Workout (pp. 64–132)

HOW I FELT: (what worked, what didn't)

_____
_____
_____
_____
_____
_____

I'M PROUD OF:

_____
_____
_____
_____
_____

DAY 5

Date:

Don't fool yourself. If you down a piece of birthday cake at the office, do you figure you'll eat less later? It's unlikely. When researchers fed 11 lean men a 250-calorie snack soon after lunch, they didn't feel more satisfied, delay dinner, or eat less later on. They simply tacked the extra calories onto their day's total. When you eat because you're hungry, blood glucose levels rise, which signals satisfaction and an end to the meal. But when you eat for other reasons, those extra calories immediately get stored as fat.

Chew on this: Researchers recently discovered that chewing sugar-free gum all day increases your metabolic rate by about 20 percent. That could burn off more than 10 pounds a year.

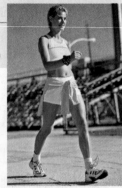

For Your Body

To walk faster, think positive. When a group of healthy people with an average age of 70 received about 30 minutes of positive subliminal messages, their walking speeds increased by 9 percent. To give yourself a similar boost when you work out, surround yourself with positive people and do things that make you feel good about yourself. Or to order our audiocassette, Prevention's Take a Walk Today, send a check for $10.95 payable to Prevention Walking Club to: Maggie Spilner, Prevention Magazine, 33 E. Minor St., Emmaus, PA 18098.

Checklist

DAILY SERVINGS

5 vegetables ☐☐☐☐☐

4 fruits ☐☐☐☐

3–6 whole ☐☐☐☐☐☐
grains

2–3 high-calcium ☐☐☐
foods

8 glasses ☐☐☐☐
of water ☐☐☐☐

1 cup of tea ☐

DAILY SUPPLEMENT NEEDS

Multivitamin/mineral ☐
100% DV for most nutrients

Vitamin C: 100–500 mg ☐
Vitamin E: 100–400 IU ☐
Calcium: 500 mg ☐

WEEKLY SERVINGS

5+ beans ☐☐☐☐☐
5 nuts ☐☐☐☐☐
2 fish ☐☐

WHAT I DID:

☐ Abs and Waist Workout (pp. 134–39)

☐ Hips, Thighs, and Buttocks Workout (pp. 140–46)

☐ Aerobic Workout (pp. 64–132)

HOW I FELT: (what worked, what didn't)

_____
_____
_____
_____
_____
_____

WHAT I ATE:

_____
_____
_____
_____
_____
_____
_____

I'M PROUD OF:

_____
_____
_____
_____
_____
_____

DAY 6

Date:

FOR THE RECORD

Uncover your emotional eating habits. Every time you eat today, write down what you ate and why you ate it. Were you hungry? Or were you mad? Or sad? Or bored? Charting your emotional eating will help you get a handle on just how much food you consume when you're not even hungry.

Brown-bag it: Dining out for lunch more than five times a week may make you eat more—nearly 300 extra calories a day—than you would if you made your own meals.

For Your Plate

Control your splurges. Successful weight loss allows, even encourages you to plan for an occasional indulgence of favorite foods. In a study of 24 obese women, the group that learned how to deal with foods they considered a problem were able to lose weight steadily and keep it off much better than those who just restricted calories, who lost initially but tended to regain the weight. Instead of saying, "I can't have potato chips," decide if you really want them. If the answer is yes, determine a reasonable amount to eat, then enjoy. If you don't see anything as forbidden, you eliminate the seduction and struggle of resisting certain foods.

Checklist

DAILY SERVINGS

5 vegetables	☐☐☐☐☐
4 fruits	☐☐☐☐
3–6 whole grains	☐☐☐☐☐☐
2–3 high-calcium foods	☐☐☐
8 glasses of water	☐☐☐☐ ☐☐☐☐
1 cup of tea	☐

DAILY SUPPLEMENT NEEDS

Multivitamin/mineral ☐
100% DV for most nutrients

Vitamin C: 100–500 mg ☐

Vitamin E: 100–400 IU ☐

Calcium: 500 mg ☐

WEEKLY SERVINGS

5+ beans	☐☐☐☐☐
5 nuts	☐☐☐☐☐
2 fish	☐☐

WHAT I DID:

☐ Abs and Waist Workout (pp. 134–39)

☐ Hips, Thighs, and Buttocks Workout (pp. 140–46)

☐ Aerobic Workout (pp. 64–132)

HOW I FELT: (what worked, what didn't)

_____
_____
_____
_____
_____
_____

WHAT I ATE:

_____
_____
_____
_____
_____
_____

I'M PROUD OF:

_____
_____
_____
_____
_____
_____

DAY 7

Date:

FOR YOUR MIND **Make toning more uplifting.** If you can't wait to be done with a toning routine, make lifting fun. If you like camaraderie, join a strength-training class at a local gym. If you prefer going solo, do your moves in front of a mirror and focus on your form. Still bored? Work out while you watch TV.

Out with the new: You could easily shed an extra 200 calories a day if you stop using the TV/VCR remote, electric can opener, riding mower, and other modern labor-saving devices.

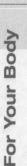
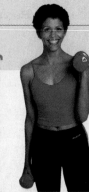

For Your Body

Hammer time. Here's a variation on the biceps curl, called the hammer curl. This exercise targets the biceps as well as the small brachialis muscles beneath the biceps, which show results fast. Start by standing upright, feet shoulder-width apart, holding a dumbbell in each hand, palms facing in. Bend your left elbow, slowly raising the dumbbell toward your left shoulder in a slow motion. Only your hand and forearm should move. Lift until the dumbbell is nearly touching your shoulder. Pause, then slowly lower. Do 8 to 12 reps per arm for 1 to 3 sets.

Checklist

DAILY SERVINGS

5 vegetables ☐☐☐☐☐

4 fruits ☐☐☐☐

3–6 whole ☐☐☐☐☐☐
grains

2–3 high-calcium ☐☐☐
foods

8 glasses ☐☐☐☐
of water ☐☐☐☐

1 cup of tea ☐

DAILY SUPPLEMENT NEEDS

Multivitamin/mineral ☐
100% DV for most nutrients

Vitamin C: 100–500 mg ☐
Vitamin E: 100–400 IU ☐
Calcium: 500 mg ☐

WEEKLY SERVINGS

5+ beans ☐☐☐☐☐
5 nuts ☐☐☐☐☐
2 fish ☐☐

WHAT I DID:

☐ Abs and Waist Workout (pp. 134–39)
☐ Hips, Thighs, and Buttocks Workout (pp. 140–46)
☐ Aerobic Workout (pp. 64–132)

HOW I FELT: (what worked, what didn't)

_____
_____
_____
_____
_____

WHAT I ATE:

_____
_____
_____
_____
_____
_____

I'M PROUD OF:

_____
_____
_____
_____
_____
_____

DAY 8

Date:

FOR THE RECORD

Check your pace. Though this may not seem to be a likely problem unless you're training for a triathlon, anyone whose heart rate is too high during exercise could be putting herself at risk for muscle and joint injuries or, in some cases, cardiovascular complications. To check your exercise intensity, take your pulse for 10 seconds. If it's higher than the recommended upper limit on the chart below, tone down your workout a bit until you're in range.

AGE	UPPER LIMIT for a 10-SECOND COUNT	UPPER LIMIT for HEART RATE (BEATS PER MINUTE)
35	22–25	130–148
40	21–24	126–144
45	21–23	123–140
50	20–23	119–136
55	19–22	116–132
60	19–21	112–128
65	18–21	109–124

For Your Plate

Burn more with breakfast. Contrary to what some folks believe, eating breakfast won't boost your metabolism, but skipping it could lead to a 5 percent drop in your resting metabolic rate. Translation: You'll burn fewer calories at rest than someone who eats three or more meals a day. That small 5 percent can add up to a 10-pound weight difference in a year.

Checklist

DAILY SERVINGS

5 vegetables ☐☐☐☐☐

4 fruits ☐☐☐☐

3–6 whole ☐☐☐☐☐☐
grains

2–3 high-calcium ☐☐☐
foods

8 glasses ☐☐☐☐
of water ☐☐☐☐

1 cup of tea ☐

DAILY SUPPLEMENT NEEDS

Multivitamin/mineral ☐
100% DV for most nutrients

Vitamin C: 100–500 mg ☐

Vitamin E: 100–400 IU ☐

Calcium: 500 mg ☐

WEEKLY SERVINGS

5+ beans ☐☐☐☐☐

5 nuts ☐☐☐☐☐

2 fish ☐☐

WHAT I DID:

☐ Abs and Waist Workout (pp. 134–39)

☐ Hips, Thighs, and Buttocks Workout (pp. 140–46)

☐ Aerobic Workout (pp. 64–132)

HOW I FELT: (what worked, what didn't)

_____
_____
_____
_____
_____
_____

WHAT I ATE:

_____
_____
_____
_____
_____
_____
_____

I'M PROUD OF:

_____
_____
_____
_____
_____
_____

DAY 9

Date:

FOR YOUR MIND

Don't be "list-less." If your resolve is already flagging, it's time to get out your pen and paper. Close your eyes and take a few minutes to revisit what has brought you to this point in your life. Write down all of the reasons you want to slim down (not the reasons others think you should). Post your list on the fridge and keep a copy in your wallet. When your motivation wanes, give it a read and congratulate yourself for choosing a healthier life.

Want proof that starch is sugar? Put a white cracker in your mouth, chew it, and hold it there. As your saliva breaks down the starch, it will start to taste sweet.

For Your Body

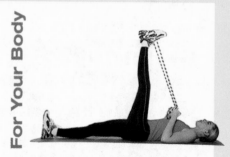

Get a leg up. If your hamstring muscles are too tight, they can pull on your pelvis, which isn't good for your back. Here's a stretch to loosen them up: Loop a towel or rope under the arch of your left foot and lie flat on your back, legs straight out on the floor. Keeping your knee straight, pull your left leg off the floor until you feel a stretch. Hold 10 to 30 seconds, then release. Keep your back pressed to the floor throughout the stretch. Repeat three times per leg; do this five or six times a week.

Checklist

DAILY SERVINGS

5 vegetables ☐☐☐☐☐

4 fruits ☐☐☐☐

3–6 whole ☐☐☐☐☐☐
grains

2–3 high-calcium ☐☐☐
foods

8 glasses ☐☐☐☐
of water ☐☐☐☐

1 cup of tea ☐

DAILY SUPPLEMENT NEEDS

Multivitamin/mineral ☐
100% DV for most nutrients

Vitamin C: 100–500 mg ☐
Vitamin E: 100–400 IU ☐
Calcium: 500 mg ☐

WEEKLY SERVINGS

5+ beans ☐☐☐☐☐
5 nuts ☐☐☐☐☐
2 fish ☐☐

WHAT I DID:

☐ Abs and Waist Workout (pp. 134–39)

☐ Hips, Thighs, and Buttocks Workout (pp. 140–46)

☐ Aerobic Workout (pp. 64–132)

HOW I FELT: (what worked, what didn't)

_____
_____
_____
_____
_____

WHAT I ATE:

_____
_____
_____
_____
_____
_____

I'M PROUD OF:

_____
_____
_____
_____
_____

DAY 10

Date:

FOR THE RECORD

Weight it out. Make sure you're not lifting too much weight . . . or too little during your strength-training workouts. If you can't do 8 repetitions at a time, the weight you are using is too heavy. If you can do 12 easily, the weight is too light.

Drop and do 10: Before you pry open that tub of ice cream, do 10 situps or pushups. Distracting yourself with something physical can put you back in touch with your body—and your goals.

For Your Plate

Slurp some soup. Having a broth-based soup at the beginning of a meal can help you eat less. In one study, three groups of women ate either a large bowl of chicken-rice soup, the same amount of chicken-rice casserole, or the casserole and a 10-ounce glass of water. In each case, the appetizer was made up of the same ingredients, but the women who ate the soup version subsequently chose lunches that were about 100 calories less than the lunches the other eaters had. Over the course of a year, that 100 fewer calories per day can add up to 10 pounds lost.

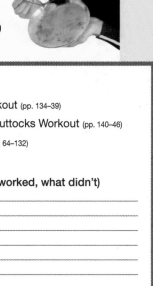

Checklist

DAILY SERVINGS

5 vegetables	☐☐☐☐☐
4 fruits	☐☐☐☐
3–6 whole grains	☐☐☐☐☐☐
2–3 high-calcium foods	☐☐☐
8 glasses of water	☐☐☐☐ ☐☐☐☐
1 cup of tea	☐

DAILY SUPPLEMENT NEEDS

Multivitamin/mineral 100% DV for most nutrients	☐
Vitamin C: 100–500 mg	☐
Vitamin E: 100–400 IU	☐
Calcium: 500 mg	☐

WEEKLY SERVINGS

5+ beans	☐☐☐☐☐
5 nuts	☐☐☐☐☐
2 fish	☐☐

WHAT I DID:

☐ Abs and Waist Workout (pp. 134–39)

☐ Hips, Thighs, and Buttocks Workout (pp. 140–46)

☐ Aerobic Workout (pp. 64–132)

HOW I FELT: (what worked, what didn't)

_____
_____
_____
_____
_____

WHAT I ATE:

_____
_____
_____
_____
_____
_____

I'M PROUD OF:

_____
_____
_____
_____
_____
_____

DAY 11

Date:

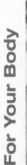

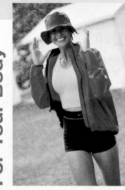

FOR YOUR MIND

Get outta here. Want to take your mind off your workout and burn more calories to boot? Move your workout outside. Exercising outdoors seems to unconsciously stimulate you to move faster, according to studies on walkers. When you're inside, you tend to focus on how miserable you are. When out of doors, you're pleasantly distracted by your surroundings. Pay attention to the sights, sounds, and aromas around you, and your workout will be done before you know it.

Juicy tidbit: A glass of 100 percent juice sometimes offers more nutrients than a single piece of fruit, but it packs none of the fiber. Also, juices tend to be higher in calories than whole fruits. Bottom line: Don't rely on juice alone to fulfill your fruit quota.

For Your Body

Adopt an all-weather policy. Don't let rain showers stop your program; it's only water! To make sure you can weather the weather, dress in garments that breathe. (Don't wear a plastic slicker; it will keep the rain out but trap sweat in.) Walk on asphalt or concrete and avoid slippery surfaces like wet grass or mud. Use a hat or visor to keep the rain off your face, and wear bright or reflective clothing so motorists can see you.

Checklist

DAILY SERVINGS

5 vegetables ☐☐☐☐☐

4 fruits ☐☐☐☐

3–6 whole grains ☐☐☐☐☐☐

2–3 high-calcium foods ☐☐☐

8 glasses of water ☐☐☐☐ ☐☐☐☐

1 cup of tea ☐

DAILY SUPPLEMENT NEEDS

Multivitamin/mineral ☐
100% DV for most nutrients

Vitamin C: 100–500 mg ☐
Vitamin E: 100–400 IU ☐
Calcium: 500 mg ☐

WEEKLY SERVINGS

5+ beans ☐☐☐☐☐
5 nuts ☐☐☐☐☐
2 fish ☐☐

WHAT I DID:

☐ Abs and Waist Workout (pp. 134–39)

☐ Hips, Thighs, and Buttocks Workout (pp. 140–46)

☐ Aerobic Workout (pp. 64–132)

HOW I FELT: (what worked, what didn't)

_____
_____
_____
_____
_____

WHAT I ATE:

_____
_____
_____
_____
_____

I'M PROUD OF:

_____
_____
_____
_____

DAY 12

Date:

FOR THE RECORD
Build a weight-loss wardrobe.

Though you may not want to revamp your whole wardrobe each time you lose 5 pounds, you'll feel better if you have a few clothes that fit. To save bucks, check out consignment shops, discount chains, and thrift stores for "temporary" clothes. Donate 'em back once you've gotten down to your goal weight.

Shoe news: If your walking or running shoes get wet, stuff them with newspaper to speed drying. Or, better yet, have a backup pair so you can alternate between them.

For Your Plate

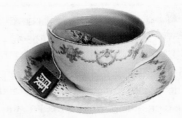

Time your tea break. If you're downing your morning multivitamin with a cup of hot tea, you may be cheating yourself. Compounds in tea called tannins, which offer protection against certain cancers and heart disease, interfere with the body's absorption of the mineral iron. That's why it's best not to drink tea within 90 minutes of taking a multi with iron or any iron supplements your doc has prescribed.

Checklist

DAILY SERVINGS

5 vegetables ☐☐☐☐☐

4 fruits ☐☐☐☐

3–6 whole ☐☐☐☐☐☐
grains

2–3 high-calcium ☐☐☐
foods

8 glasses ☐☐☐☐
of water ☐☐☐☐

1 cup of tea ☐

DAILY SUPPLEMENT NEEDS

Multivitamin/mineral ☐
100% DV for most nutrients

Vitamin C: 100–500 mg ☐

Vitamin E: 100–400 IU ☐

Calcium: 500 mg ☐

WEEKLY SERVINGS

5+ beans ☐☐☐☐☐

5 nuts ☐☐☐☐☐

2 fish ☐☐

WHAT I DID:

☐ Abs and Waist Workout (pp. 134–39)

☐ Hips, Thighs, and Buttocks Workout (pp. 140–46)

☐ Aerobic Workout (pp. 64–132)

HOW I FELT: (what worked, what didn't)

_____
_____
_____
_____
_____
_____

WHAT I ATE:

_____
_____
_____
_____
_____
_____

I'M PROUD OF:

_____
_____
_____
_____
_____

Date:

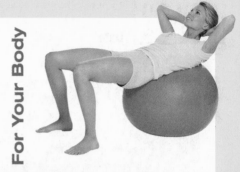

For Your Body

 Take a deep breath. Stress raises levels of cortisol, a hormone that seems to direct fat to your belly. To soothe your mind (and keep your tummy toned), take 5 minutes a day to focus on slow, deep breathing, while repeating the word "one" as you exhale.

Listen up. If you strap on a personal CD player or other stereo while exercising outdoors, wear the headphones slightly in front of or behind your ears, and keep the volume low. This allows you to better hear approaching cars, bikes, or unsavory characters—and to act quickly when necessary.

Get on the ball. Here's a great way to increase the payoff of your ab workout: Use an exercise ball. Because it's more difficult to do crunches on the ball, you don't have to do as many before you see results. Aim for 10 to 12 reps, two or three times a week. Here's the technique: Position the ball so it's supporting your back. Put your feet flat on the floor. Start with your arms extended in front of you, then slowly curl up. Hold, then lower. For more difficulty, place your hands behind your head.

Checklist

DAILY SERVINGS

5 vegetables ☐☐☐☐☐

4 fruits ☐☐☐☐

3–6 whole ☐☐☐☐☐☐
grains

2–3 high-calcium ☐☐☐
foods

8 glasses ☐☐☐☐
of water ☐☐☐☐

1 cup of tea ☐

DAILY SUPPLEMENT NEEDS

Multivitamin/mineral ☐
100% DV for most nutrients

Vitamin C: 100–500 mg ☐
Vitamin E: 100–400 IU ☐
Calcium: 500 mg ☐

WEEKLY SERVINGS

5+ beans ☐☐☐☐☐
5 nuts ☐☐☐☐☐
2 fish ☐☐

WHAT I DID:
☐ Abs and Waist Workout (pp. 134–39)
☐ Hips, Thighs, and Buttocks Workout (pp. 140–46)
☐ Aerobic Workout (pp. 64–132)

HOW I FELT: (what worked, what didn't)

WHAT I ATE:

I'M PROUD OF:

DAY 14

Date:

FOR THE RECORD **Park far away.** If you're always jockeying for the space that's closest to the door, you're doing yourself a disservice. It's less stressful to park farther away instead of contending for a close spot, and it also adds a little extra calorie burn to your day. You can even use your car's odometer to clock the distance from the farthest space to the door, and count that "mileage" toward your workout.

Talk back. Pay attention when negative thoughts pop into your head. Every time your internal voice starts saying, "I'm too fat" or "I can't do it," answer back: "That's enough. I can do whatever I put my mind to."

For Your Plate

Eat more meals. If you starve yourself all day and then scarf down a big dinner, you're not keeping your body consistently fueled, which can leave you dragging. What's more, if you consume 50 grams or more of fat at one sitting (which isn't hard to do at one big meal), your arteries lose flexibility for the next 4 hours— a period of time that one researcher has described as a "heart attack danger zone." Aim for no fewer than three meals a day, or a series of mini-meals throughout the day.

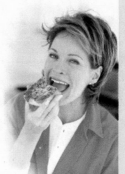

Checklist

DAILY SERVINGS

5 vegetables ☐☐☐☐☐

4 fruits ☐☐☐☐

3–6 whole grains ☐☐☐☐☐☐

2–3 high-calcium foods ☐☐☐

8 glasses of water ☐☐☐☐ ☐☐☐☐

1 cup of tea ☐

DAILY SUPPLEMENT NEEDS

Multivitamin/mineral ☐
100% DV for most nutrients

Vitamin C: 100–500 mg ☐
Vitamin E: 100–400 IU ☐
Calcium: 500 mg ☐

WEEKLY SERVINGS

5+ beans ☐☐☐☐☐
5 nuts ☐☐☐☐☐
2 fish ☐☐

WHAT I DID:

☐ Abs and Waist Workout (pp. 134–39)

☐ Hips, Thighs, and Buttocks Workout (pp. 140–46)

☐ Aerobic Workout (pp. 64–132)

HOW I FELT: (what worked, what didn't)

_____
_____
_____
_____
_____

WHAT I ATE:

_____
_____
_____
_____
_____

I'M PROUD OF:

_____
_____
_____
_____
_____

DAY 15

Date:

FOR YOUR MIND

Go digital. Keeping tabs on your weight by using a scale can help you chart your progress—and nip any unexpected "regains" in the bud. But if you have one of those scales with a drifting needle, it can be tough to tell just what number to record in your journal. Trading up to a digital scale can help take the guesswork out of weekly weigh-ins.

Get more fiber. Sprinkle high-fiber ground flaxseed on your cereal in the morning to help curb your appetite. You can also add this grain (available in health food stores) to yogurt or bread and muffin mixes.

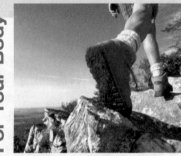

For Your Body

Pack it in. To boost your calorie burn and have more fun, too, do your walk on some nature trails and carry a fanny pack or backpack. Pretend you're an explorer, and take a magnifying glass, a bird guidebook, binoculars, a camera, a novel, a bottle of water, and a plastic bag or container for rocks or leaves or whatever you collect on your walk. While an hour of trail walking with no extra weight burns 258 calories, carrying an extra 5 pounds burns 272. Just don't overdo it: Even a little extra weight can feel like a ton when you're not used to it.

Checklist

DAILY SERVINGS

5 vegetables ☐☐☐☐☐

4 fruits ☐☐☐☐

3–6 whole grains ☐☐☐☐☐☐

2–3 high-calcium foods ☐☐☐

8 glasses of water ☐☐☐☐ ☐☐☐☐

1 cup of tea ☐

DAILY SUPPLEMENT NEEDS

Multivitamin/mineral ☐
100% DV for most nutrients

Vitamin C: 100–500 mg ☐
Vitamin E: 100–400 IU ☐
Calcium: 500 mg ☐

WEEKLY SERVINGS

5+ beans ☐☐☐☐☐
5 nuts ☐☐☐☐☐
2 fish ☐☐

WHAT I DID:

☐ Abs and Waist Workout (pp. 134–39)

☐ Hips, Thighs, and Buttocks Workout (pp. 140–46)

☐ Aerobic Workout (pp. 64–132)

HOW I FELT: (what worked, what didn't)

_____
_____
_____
_____
_____
_____

WHAT I ATE:

_____
_____
_____
_____
_____
_____

I'M PROUD OF:

_____
_____
_____
_____
_____
_____

DAY 16

Date:

FOR THE RECORD

Weigh your clothes. That's right . . . you may be surprised to find that those jeans, that sweater, and those sneakers all add up to a couple of pounds. For the most accurate weigh-ins, step on the scale in only your birthday suit every time. That way, a "heavy" outfit won't budge the number upward and make you feel like a failure.

Give 'em the boot. If you're trail walking today, trade your walking shoes for some good hiking boots. Even if you're fit and an avid walker, your feet will feel every rock and pebble in regular shoes.

For Your Plate

Eat before or after. Think you'll burn more calories if you exercise on an empty stomach? Sorry, but that's an old wives' tale. Whether your body gets its energy from "new" food or stored fat, it will replenish its energy stores at some point. The key to burning off fat is to exercise regularly so that you'll burn off more total calories than you consume in a day.

Checklist

DAILY SERVINGS

5 vegetables	☐☐☐☐☐ •
4 fruits	☐☐☐☐
3–6 whole grains	☐☐☐☐☐☐
2–3 high-calcium foods	☐☐☐
8 glasses of water	☐☐☐☐ ☐☐☐☐
1 cup of tea	☐

DAILY SUPPLEMENT NEEDS

Multivitamin/mineral 100% DV for most nutrients	☐
Vitamin C: 100–500 mg	☐
Vitamin E: 100–400 IU	☐
Calcium: 500 mg	☐

WEEKLY SERVINGS

5+ beans	☐☐☐☐☐
5 nuts	☐☐☐☐☐
2 fish	☐☐

WHAT I DID:

☐ Abs and Waist Workout (pp. 134–39)

☐ Hips, Thighs, and Buttocks Workout (pp. 140–46)

☐ Aerobic Workout (pp. 64–132)

HOW I FELT: (what worked, what didn't)

_____
_____
_____
_____
_____
_____

WHAT I ATE:

_____
_____
_____
_____
_____

I'M PROUD OF:

_____
_____
_____
_____

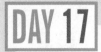

DAY 17   Date:

 FOR YOUR MIND **Avoid popcorn overload.** If you tend to snack too much at the movies, choose scary shows over chick flicks. You're less likely to eat when you're fearful and more likely to eat when you're happy (or angry).

Don't pump up iron with pills. Some research suggests that too much iron may raise the risk of heart disease and colon cancer, so don't take iron pills unless your doctor has tested you for deficiency and recommends supplementation.

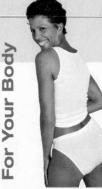

For Your Body

Don't choose cotton. When exercising in cool weather, it's best to wear undergarments made from fabrics like polypropylene, CoolMax, Dri-FIT, or Capilene, which help wick moisture away from your skin. In fact, wearing panties and bras made from wicking fabrics can keep you drier and more comfortable all year round, possibly even reducing your risk for vaginal infections. You'll find these high-tech undies at most sporting goods and department stores or in catalogs such as L. L. Bean, Title Nine Sports, and Campmor.

Checklist

DAILY SERVINGS

5 vegetables ☐☐☐☐☐

4 fruits ☐☐☐☐

3–6 whole grains ☐☐☐☐☐☐

2–3 high-calcium foods ☐☐☐

8 glasses of water ☐☐☐☐ ☐☐☐☐

1 cup of tea ☐

DAILY SUPPLEMENT NEEDS

Multivitamin/mineral ☐
100% DV for most nutrients

Vitamin C: 100–500 mg ☐
Vitamin E: 100–400 IU ☐
Calcium: 500 mg ☐

WEEKLY SERVINGS

5+ beans ☐☐☐☐☐
5 nuts ☐☐☐☐☐
2 fish ☐☐

WHAT I DID:
☐ Abs and Waist Workout (pp. 134–39)
☐ Hips, Thighs, and Buttocks Workout (pp. 140–46)
☐ Aerobic Workout (pp. 64–132)

HOW I FELT: (what worked, what didn't)
_____
_____
_____
_____
_____
_____

WHAT I ATE:
_____
_____
_____
_____
_____

I'M PROUD OF:
_____
_____
_____
_____
_____

DAY 18

Date:

FOR THE RECORD

Skim the fat. You're probably consuming more pure fat from cooking oils, butter, and margarine than you realize. Even healthier choices like olive oil can add up. Today, tally the calories and grams you eat from pure fats. If the total is high, try cutting back and substituting fat-free margarine sprays or a mist of olive oil where you'd normally butter things up.

Walk while you talk. Put a little calorie burn into your next conversation: While you're on the cordless phone, do laundry (68 calories), set the table (85 calories), or water the plants (102 calories).

For Your Plate

Just spray it. Your olive oil, that is. Using an olive oil sprayer such as Misto distributes your oil better so you can use less. A 2-second spritz evenly covers food with about ½ teaspoon of oil, compared with the 2 or 3 teaspoons you'd likely use if you drizzled it straight out of the bottle. Calorie savings: 100 per use.

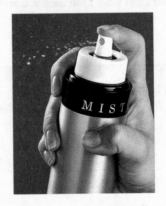

Checklist

DAILY SERVINGS

5 vegetables ☐☐☐☐☐

4 fruits ☐☐☐☐

3–6 whole grains ☐☐☐☐☐☐

2–3 high-calcium foods ☐☐☐

8 glasses of water ☐☐☐☐ ☐☐☐☐

1 cup of tea ☐

DAILY SUPPLEMENT NEEDS

Multivitamin/mineral ☐
100% DV for most nutrients

Vitamin C: 100–500 mg ☐

Vitamin E: 100–400 IU ☐

Calcium: 500 mg ☐

WEEKLY SERVINGS

5+ beans ☐☐☐☐☐

5 nuts ☐☐☐☐☐

2 fish ☐☐

WHAT I DID:

☐ Abs and Waist Workout (pp. 134–39)

☐ Hips, Thighs, and Buttocks Workout (pp. 140–46)

☐ Aerobic Workout (pp. 64–132)

HOW I FELT: (what worked, what didn't)

_____
_____
_____
_____
_____

WHAT I ATE:

_____
_____
_____
_____
_____
_____

I'M PROUD OF:

_____
_____
_____
_____
_____
_____

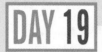

DAY 19

Date:

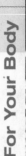

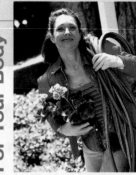

FOR YOUR MIND

Play road games. If your walking workout is getting to be lame, make it a game. Walk for as long as it takes to spot three red cars, then do some stretches. Look for all the letters of the alphabet (in order) on people's mailboxes, street signs, and so forth. Or pick up the pace until you reach the next stop sign, then slow it down until you see another one.

Heat things up. Adding a hot chile pepper to your meal may stop your eating sooner. Zesty foods are more satisfying—and you simply can't handle eating as much of them.

For Your Body

Do a backyard workout. It'll take more than pulling a few weeds, but you can burn more calories in your yard than in the gym. When researchers tested a 40-year-old woman, they found that she burned nearly 30 percent more calories while working outdoors (sawing, carrying, and piling debris) than she did during a step aerobics class! What's more, though both workouts lasted an hour, she spent 44 minutes working in her target heart rate zone while in the garden, but just 24 minutes in the zone during aerobics class. Her calorie burn for an hour of heavy gardening? A whopping 392!

Checklist

DAILY SERVINGS

5 vegetables ☐☐☐☐☐

4 fruits ☐☐☐☐

3–6 whole grains ☐☐☐☐☐☐

2–3 high-calcium foods ☐☐☐

8 glasses of water ☐☐☐☐ ☐☐☐☐

1 cup of tea ☐

DAILY SUPPLEMENT NEEDS

Multivitamin/mineral ☐
100% DV for most nutrients

Vitamin C: 100–500 mg ☐

Vitamin E: 100–400 IU ☐

Calcium: 500 mg ☐

WEEKLY SERVINGS

5+ beans ☐☐☐☐☐

5 nuts ☐☐☐☐☐

2 fish ☐☐

WHAT I DID:

☐ Abs and Waist Workout (pp. 134–39)

☐ Hips, Thighs, and Buttocks Workout (pp. 140–46)

☐ Aerobic Workout (pp. 64–132)

HOW I FELT: (what worked, what didn't)

_____
_____
_____
_____
_____

WHAT I ATE:

_____
_____
_____
_____
_____
_____
_____

I'M PROUD OF:

_____
_____
_____
_____
_____

DAY 20

Date:

FOR THE RECORD

Clean up, trim down. Generally speaking, ½ hour of housework burns between 90 and 150 calories. And that's nothing to sneeze at (except when you're dusting). Today, tally up the minutes you spend slaving over a hot stove and otherwise keeping house, and add that to your day's calorie burn. It's like adding an extra workout to your day.

Keep a spare in the trunk. A spare pair of walking shoes and socks, that is. This way, you can slip them on and take a stroll whenever opportunity arises, say, the next time you drive to a meeting only to find out it's postponed for an hour.

For Your Plate

Can the preserves. If you're counting on jelly, jam, or preserves as a serving of fruit, think again. These toast toppers contain lots of refined sugar, which your body doesn't need. Plus, the canning process eliminates much of the fruit's fiber. A better substitute when fresh fruit is scarce (or you just haven't made it to the store this week) is canned or frozen fruit that doesn't have heavy syrup or sugar added.

Checklist

DAILY SERVINGS

5 vegetables ☐☐☐☐☐

4 fruits ☐☐☐☐

3–6 whole ☐☐☐☐☐☐
grains

2–3 high-calcium ☐☐☐
foods

8 glasses ☐☐☐☐
of water ☐☐☐☐

1 cup of tea ☐

DAILY SUPPLEMENT NEEDS

Multivitamin/mineral ☐
100% DV for most nutrients

Vitamin C: 100–500 mg ☐

Vitamin E: 100–400 IU ☐

Calcium: 500 mg ☐

WEEKLY SERVINGS

5+ beans ☐☐☐☐☐

5 nuts ☐☐☐☐☐

2 fish ☐☐

WHAT I DID:

☐ Abs and Waist Workout (pp. 134–39)

☐ Hips, Thighs, and Buttocks Workout (pp. 140–46)

☐ Aerobic Workout (pp. 64–132)

HOW I FELT: (what worked, what didn't)

_____
_____
_____
_____
_____
_____

WHAT I ATE:

_____
_____
_____
_____
_____

I'M PROUD OF:

_____
_____
_____
_____
_____

DAY 21

Date:

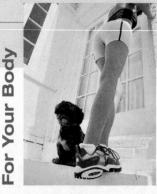

For Your Body

FOR YOUR MIND

Don't stray while you're away.
When you vacation, it can be tough to curb the urge to splurge—especially when you're faced with lots of new and naughty foods. Every time you eat, consider it a challenge to have at least one fruit or vegetable with each meal. Keep track of each time you eat a healthful food, and set aside a dollar. On the last day of the trip, count your earnings, then buy yourself a souvenir!

Mineral mistake. Taking your 500-milligram calcium supplement with a glass of calcium-fortified OJ? Don't do it! Your body can only absorb 500 milligrams of this mineral at a time. For best results, divvy up your doses so you get no more than 500 milligrams at one sitting.

Test your Achilles. Tight calf muscles can triple your risk of developing Achilles tendon problems, says a recent study. To test your flexibility, sit in a chair with your bare feet flat on the floor. Without flexing your foot, lift one leg so it's straight out in front of you and parallel to the floor. Your foot should be at a 90-degree angle, toes pointing skyward. Now flex your foot, bringing your toes toward your head. If you can't flex more than the initial 90-degree angle, your calf is tight and you should do more stretches. Test both legs, since one may be tighter than the other.

Checklist

DAILY SERVINGS		DAILY SUPPLEMENT NEEDS	
5 vegetables	❑❑❑❑❑	Multivitamin/mineral ❑ 100% DV for most nutrients	
4 fruits	❑❑❑❑	Vitamin C: 100–500 mg ❑	
3–6 whole grains	❑❑❑❑❑❑	Vitamin E: 100–400 IU ❑	
2–3 high-calcium foods	❑❑❑	Calcium: 500 mg ❑	
8 glasses of water	❑❑❑❑ ❑❑❑❑	**WEEKLY SERVINGS**	
1 cup of tea	❑	5+ beans	❑❑❑❑❑
		5 nuts	❑❑❑❑❑
		2 fish	❑❑

WHAT I DID:
- ❑ Abs and Waist Workout (pp. 134–39)
- ❑ Hips, Thighs, and Buttocks Workout (pp. 140–46)
- ❑ Aerobic Workout (pp. 64–132)

HOW I FELT: (what worked, what didn't)
_____
_____
_____
_____
_____

WHAT I ATE:
_____
_____
_____
_____
_____
_____

I'M PROUD OF:
_____
_____
_____
_____
_____

DAY 22

Date:

FOR THE RECORD

Count to 10,000. Clip a pedometer to your waistband in the morning. It can make you more active—even on days when you don't exercise. Aim for 10,000 steps, and you'll find yourself sitting less and walking more. The simplest and most accurate brand of pedometer we found is New Lifestyles' SW-401 Digiwalker Pedometer by Yamax. To order or find a store near you, visit the Web site www.digiwalker.com. Cost: about $30.

Way to go! Go ahead—compliment yourself. You should treat you as you treat those you love. Focus on successes, not failures, and give yourself a pat on the back each day.

For Your Plate

Opt for lobster. Here's one rich dish you can splurge on anytime. Sweet Maine lobster has only 83 calories in 3 ounces—even less than skinless turkey breast! But skip the butter dipping sauce—this super seafood doesn't need it and neither do you.

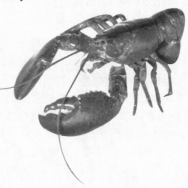

Checklist

DAILY SERVINGS

5 vegetables ☐☐☐☐☐

4 fruits ☐☐☐☐

3–6 whole grains ☐☐☐☐☐☐

2–3 high-calcium foods ☐☐☐

8 glasses of water ☐☐☐☐ ☐☐☐☐

1 cup of tea ☐

DAILY SUPPLEMENT NEEDS

Multivitamin/mineral ☐
100% DV for most nutrients

Vitamin C: 100–500 mg ☐

Vitamin E: 100–400 IU ☐

Calcium: 500 mg ☐

WEEKLY SERVINGS

5+ beans ☐☐☐☐☐

5 nuts ☐☐☐☐☐

2 fish ☐☐

WHAT I DID:

☐ Abs and Waist Workout (pp. 134–39)

☐ Hips, Thighs, and Buttocks Workout (pp. 140–46)

☐ Aerobic Workout (pp. 64–132)

HOW I FELT: (what worked, what didn't)

_____
_____
_____
_____
_____
_____

WHAT I ATE:

_____
_____
_____
_____
_____
_____

I'M PROUD OF:

_____
_____
_____
_____
_____

DAY 23

Date: _____

FOR YOUR MIND

Spread the word. According to a University of Pittsburgh study, folks who received the support of friends and family during their weight-loss programs have a 95 percent chance of slimming down successfully. What's more, they're twice as likely to keep off the extra weight.

Fine-print pitfalls. Be sure to read food labels closely, especially for snack foods and beverages. At a quick glance, that candy bar appears to contain 220 calories. But a closer look may reveal that it provides two or more servings, which more than doubles those calories.

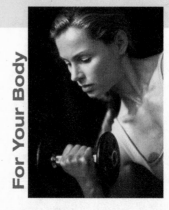

For Your Body

Target practice. Want to lose weight in one particular area? Sorry, but doing exercises that "target" that zone won't trim the fat from that area alone. Fat comes off from head to toe, so an overall aerobic program is what you really need to help burn off the fat that's covering your problem areas. And once you burn away the fat, those weight-lifting exercises you're doing will help define and strengthen the muscles you've exposed.

Checklist

DAILY SERVINGS

5 vegetables ☐☐☐☐☐

4 fruits ☐☐☐☐

3–6 whole grains ☐☐☐☐☐☐

2–3 high-calcium foods ☐☐☐

8 glasses of water ☐☐☐☐ ☐☐☐☐

1 cup of tea ☐

DAILY SUPPLEMENT NEEDS

Multivitamin/mineral ☐
100% DV for most nutrients

Vitamin C: 100–500 mg ☐
Vitamin E: 100–400 IU ☐
Calcium: 500 mg ☐

WEEKLY SERVINGS

5+ beans ☐☐☐☐☐
5 nuts ☐☐☐☐☐
2 fish ☐☐

WHAT I DID:

☐ Abs and Waist Workout (pp. 134–39)
☐ Hips, Thighs, and Buttocks Workout (pp. 140–46)
☐ Aerobic Workout (pp. 64–132)

HOW I FELT: (what worked, what didn't)

_____
_____
_____
_____
_____

WHAT I ATE:

_____
_____
_____
_____
_____

I'M PROUD OF:

_____
_____
_____
_____
_____

DAY 24

Date:

FOR THE RECORD

Keep the scale moving. Time to recheck your calorie count today. It's easy to forget exactly what and how much you're eating. If you've been exercising faithfully but aren't losing any more weight, chances are you're not eating as healthfully as you were when you started this program. Or maybe you're just in such great shape that you need to work out for a few extra minutes each day or increase the intensity. (Don't change both duration and intensity at the same time, or you could wind up injuring yourself.) Reevaluating your program can keep you on track and improve your results.

For Your Plate

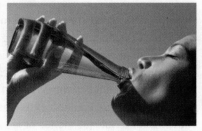

Supersize your H$_2$O. If you want to guzzle a big drink, make it a water. Dehydration can slow your metabolism by 3 percent, making you burn fewer calories throughout the day.

A dab'll do ya. Use a napkin to blot the grease off two slices of pizza, and you'll lose about a teaspoon of oil (that's 40 calories and 4.5 grams of fat).

Checklist

DAILY SERVINGS

5 vegetables ☐☐☐☐☐

4 fruits ☐☐☐☐

3–6 whole grains ☐☐☐☐☐☐

2–3 high-calcium foods ☐☐☐

8 glasses of water ☐☐☐☐ ☐☐☐☐

1 cup of tea ☐

DAILY SUPPLEMENT NEEDS

Multivitamin/mineral ☐
100% DV for most nutrients

Vitamin C: 100–500 mg ☐

Vitamin E: 100–400 IU ☐

Calcium: 500 mg ☐

WEEKLY SERVINGS

5+ beans ☐☐☐☐☐

5 nuts ☐☐☐☐☐

2 fish ☐☐

WHAT I DID:

☐ Abs and Waist Workout (pp. 134–39)

☐ Hips, Thighs, and Buttocks Workout (pp. 140–46)

☐ Aerobic Workout (pp. 64–132)

HOW I FELT: (what worked, what didn't)

_____
_____
_____
_____
_____
_____

WHAT I ATE:

_____
_____
_____
_____
_____
_____

I'M PROUD OF:

_____
_____
_____
_____
_____

DAY 25

Date:

FOR YOUR MIND

Win him over. If your mate still isn't working out with you, here's one way to give him a nudge: Tell him exercise can improve his love life! Men with large waistlines (42 inches or more) were 1½ times more likely to have erection problems than men with smaller waists (35 inches or less). And the most active men—regardless of waist size—had a 40 percent lower risk of such problems.

Take a powder: Want a quick way to freshen your hair after a lunchtime workout? Sprinkle talc-free baby powder on your roots. Only use a little if you have dark hair, and work it through well.

For Your Body

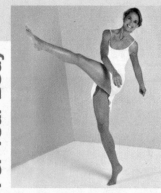

Raise prized calves. Ten million dancers can't be wrong: For shapely calves, heel raises are the best exercise you can do, and you can do them anywhere. Even better, the results are rapid. Here's the skinny: Stand with your feet about hip-width apart. If necessary, hold on to a chair for balance. Rise up slowly onto your toes. Hold, then slowly lower. To increase the difficulty, try doing one leg at a time or hold dumbbells.

Checklist

DAILY SERVINGS

5 vegetables	☐☐☐☐☐
4 fruits	☐☐☐☐
3–6 whole grains	☐☐☐☐☐☐
2–3 high-calcium foods	☐☐☐
8 glasses of water	☐☐☐☐ ☐☐☐☐
1 cup of tea	☐

DAILY SUPPLEMENT NEEDS

Multivitamin/mineral ☐
100% DV for most nutrients

Vitamin C: 100–500 mg ☐
Vitamin E: 100–400 IU ☐
Calcium: 500 mg ☐

WEEKLY SERVINGS

5+ beans	☐☐☐☐☐
5 nuts	☐☐☐☐☐
2 fish	☐☐

WHAT I DID:

☐ Abs and Waist Workout (pp. 134–39)
☐ Hips, Thighs, and Buttocks Workout (pp. 140–46)
☐ Aerobic Workout (pp. 64–132)

HOW I FELT: (what worked, what didn't)

_____
_____
_____
_____
_____
_____

WHAT I ATE:

_____
_____
_____
_____
_____
_____

I'M PROUD OF:

_____
_____
_____
_____
_____
_____

DAY 26

Date:

FOR THE RECORD

Plan in tandem. Sit down with your husband (or a friend or relative you want to work out with) and list activities he likes, then do those things together. In a 6-week study, people who felt they had a choice exercised twice as much as those who felt the choice was made for them. Your relationship and your bodies will benefit from the workout time together.

Buy premeasured portions. If you snack on some M&Ms each day, buy the tiny bags instead of grabbing a handful from the jumbo bag. You'll do better with portion control if your portions are already measured for you.

For Your Plate

Follow the 200 rule. Believe it or not, it's okay to indulge in 200 calories' worth of relatively "naughty" foods like chocolate each day. Food is psychologically satisfying and should remain that way even when you're trying to lose weight. Just be sure you substitute that 200 calories instead of adding it to what you eat. And keep the rest of your diet nutritious.

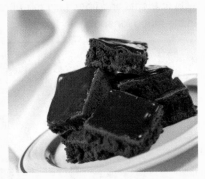

Checklist

DAILY SERVINGS

5 vegetables ☐☐☐☐☐

4 fruits ☐☐☐☐

3–6 whole ☐☐☐☐☐☐
grains

2–3 high-calcium ☐☐☐
foods

8 glasses ☐☐☐☐
of water ☐☐☐☐

1 cup of tea ☐

DAILY SUPPLEMENT NEEDS

Multivitamin/mineral ☐
100% DV for most nutrients

Vitamin C: 100–500 mg ☐
Vitamin E: 100–400 IU ☐
Calcium: 500 mg ☐

WEEKLY SERVINGS

5+ beans ☐☐☐☐☐
5 nuts ☐☐☐☐☐
2 fish ☐☐

WHAT I DID:

☐ Abs and Waist Workout (pp. 134–39)

☐ Hips, Thighs, and Buttocks Workout (pp. 140–46)

☐ Aerobic Workout (pp. 64–132)

HOW I FELT: (what worked, what didn't)

_____
_____
_____
_____
_____
_____
_____

WHAT I ATE:

_____
_____
_____
_____
_____
_____

I'M PROUD OF:

_____
_____
_____
_____
_____
_____

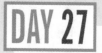

DAY 27

Date:

FOR YOUR MIND

Tame sugar addiction. Having trouble tempering your sweet tooth? Though you can't be addicted to sugar in the same way that people get addicted to drugs, sugar does trigger the release of opiates in the mind, which makes you feel good. Unfortunately, sugar also brings with it empty calories. To get that sweet-thing "high" along with nutrients and fiber, turn to fruit when you're in the mood for something sugary.

Pack a snack: Whenever you travel—especially if you don't know what the food offerings will be—take along some healthy eats. Or find a mini-mart along the way and get some fresh fruit, reduced-fat cheese, whole grain crackers, and bottled water.

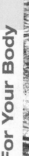
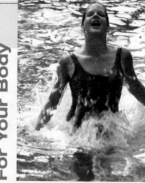

For Your Body

Get in the swim. Want to target all of your muscles at once? Hop in the pool. Swimming laps works your upper body, lower body, and even your abs and back. Swimming is also low-impact, which means it's less likely to lead to injury. The resistance of the water strengthens your muscles, and the movement gets your blood pumping, thereby strengthening your heart. If you use swimming as your main form of exercise, balance it with some weight-bearing exercise like walking, running, tennis, or weight lifting to help keep your bones strong.

Checklist

DAILY SERVINGS

5 vegetables ☐☐☐☐☐

4 fruits ☐☐☐☐

3–6 whole ☐☐☐☐☐☐
grains

2–3 high-calcium ☐☐☐
foods

8 glasses ☐☐☐☐
of water ☐☐☐☐

1 cup of tea ☐

DAILY SUPPLEMENT NEEDS

Multivitamin/mineral ☐
100% DV for most nutrients

Vitamin C: 100–500 mg ☐

Vitamin E: 100–400 IU ☐

Calcium: 500 mg ☐

WEEKLY SERVINGS

5+ beans ☐☐☐☐☐
5 nuts ☐☐☐☐☐
2 fish ☐☐

WHAT I DID:

☐ Abs and Waist Workout (pp. 134–39)

☐ Hips, Thighs, and Buttocks Workout (pp. 140–46)

☐ Aerobic Workout (pp. 64–132)

HOW I FELT: (what worked, what didn't)

_____
_____
_____
_____
_____
_____

WHAT I ATE:

_____
_____
_____
_____
_____

I'M PROUD OF:

_____
_____
_____
_____
_____

DAY 28

Date:

FOR THE RECORD — Is your medicine making you fat?

Certain drugs, including antihistamines, diabetes medications, psychiatric medications, and steroid hormones can lead to weight gain. Some stimulate appetite, others cause you to retain nutrients, calories, or fluid. If you suspect your medication may be causing you to gain weight, talk with your doctor about modifying your prescription.

Morning starter: This morning, top your whole grain bagel with 2 tablespoons of reduced-fat ricotta cheese instead of cream cheese. You'll get half the calories, one-third the fat, and five times the calcium, a mineral that may assist weight loss.

For Your Plate

Whip it up. Surprise! One tablespoon of whipped cream has only 8 calories. Plop a big tennis-ball-size dollop on a cup of strawberries for a satisfying and sweet 110-calorie dessert!

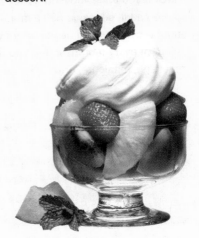

Checklist

DAILY SERVINGS

5 vegetables ☐☐☐☐☐

4 fruits ☐☐☐☐

3–6 whole grains ☐☐☐☐☐☐

2–3 high-calcium foods ☐☐☐

8 glasses of water ☐☐☐☐ ☐☐☐☐

1 cup of tea ☐

DAILY SUPPLEMENT NEEDS

Multivitamin/mineral ☐
100% DV for most nutrients

Vitamin C: 100–500 mg ☐

Vitamin E: 100–400 IU ☐

Calcium: 500 mg ☐

WEEKLY SERVINGS

5+ beans ☐☐☐☐☐

5 nuts ☐☐☐☐☐

2 fish ☐☐

WHAT I DID:

☐ Abs and Waist Workout (pp. 134–39)

☐ Hips, Thighs, and Buttocks Workout (pp. 140–46)

☐ Aerobic Workout (pp. 64–132)

HOW I FELT: (what worked, what didn't)

_____
_____
_____
_____
_____
_____

WHAT I ATE:

_____
_____
_____
_____
_____

I'M PROUD OF:

_____
_____
_____
_____
_____
_____

DAY 29

Date: _____

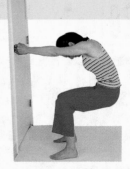

For Your Body

FOR YOUR MIND

Motivate with money. Every time you work out, put a dollar (or whatever amount you decide on) in a jar. Have your spouse match your donation, if he'll agree to it. Or if you think you'll do better with negative reinforcement, set aside $30 a month, and deduct a buck every time you don't work out. On the first of every month, spend your earnings on a massage, manicure, or another healthy reward.

The fiber/fat connection: If you double your usual fiber intake from 14 grams to about 30 grams, you'll absorb almost 120 fewer calories a day. That's 13 pounds a year!

Do a whole-body stretch. To quickly target most of the body's major muscle groups, do this hamstring stretch: Hold on to a doorknob or something sturdy. Your feet should be shoulder-width apart, toes pointing forward. Slowly sit back into a squat, keeping your knees over your ankles. Lower yourself as far as is comfortable. Slowly drop your chin to your chest and round out your back. Hold as you take six to eight slow breaths. Slowly release and stand up.

Checklist

DAILY SERVINGS

5 vegetables ☐☐☐☐☐

4 fruits ☐☐☐☐

3–6 whole grains ☐☐☐☐☐

2–3 high-calcium foods ☐☐☐

8 glasses of water ☐☐☐☐ ☐☐☐☐

1 cup of tea ☐

DAILY SUPPLEMENT NEEDS

Multivitamin/mineral ☐
  100% DV for most nutrients

Vitamin C: 100–500 mg ☐

Vitamin E: 100–400 IU ☐

Calcium: 500 mg ☐

WEEKLY SERVINGS

5+ beans ☐☐☐☐☐

5 nuts ☐☐☐☐☐

2 fish ☐☐

WHAT I DID:

☐ Abs and Waist Workout (pp. 134–39)

☐ Hips, Thighs, and Buttocks Workout (pp. 140–46)

☐ Aerobic Workout (pp. 64–132)

HOW I FELT: (what worked, what didn't)

_____
_____
_____
_____
_____
_____

WHAT I ATE:

_____
_____
_____
_____
_____

I'M PROUD OF:

_____
_____
_____
_____

DAY 30

Date:

FOR THE RECORD

Do one more checkup. You've likely found a rhythm by now, working out at basically the same time each day, showering, changing, whatever. Now it's time to look at the days when working out *doesn't* happen. What is it that throws you off track? Take steps to make sure such derailments won't happen in the future. For instance, if unexpected phone calls wreck your workouts some evenings, take the receiver off the hook till you're done. Hire a babysitter if you can't count on your husband to get home from work in time for you to join your running group. You get the picture.

For Your Plate

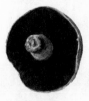

Try some mushroom magic. Brushed with olive oil and grilled or roasted, portobello mushrooms taste so rich that you can substitute them for meat. Plus, they have just 26 calories in 3.5 ounces!

Take a stretch break: Military recruits who increased their flexibility had 50 percent fewer injuries than those who were less limber. Stretch three times a day, in addition to your exercise routine.

Checklist

DAILY SERVINGS

5 vegetables ☐☐☐☐☐

4 fruits ☐☐☐☐

3–6 whole grains ☐☐☐☐☐

2–3 high-calcium foods ☐☐☐

8 glasses of water ☐☐☐☐ ☐☐☐☐

1 cup of tea ☐

DAILY SUPPLEMENT NEEDS

Multivitamin/mineral ☐
100% DV for most nutrients

Vitamin C: 100–500 mg ☐

Vitamin E: 100–400 IU ☐

Calcium: 500 mg ☐

WEEKLY SERVINGS

5+ beans ☐☐☐☐☐

5 nuts ☐☐☐☐☐

2 fish ☐☐

WHAT I DID:

☐ Abs and Waist Workout (pp. 134–39)

☐ Hips, Thighs, and Buttocks Workout (pp. 140–46)

☐ Aerobic Workout (pp. 64–132)

HOW I FELT: (what worked, what didn't)

WHAT I ATE:

I'M PROUD OF:

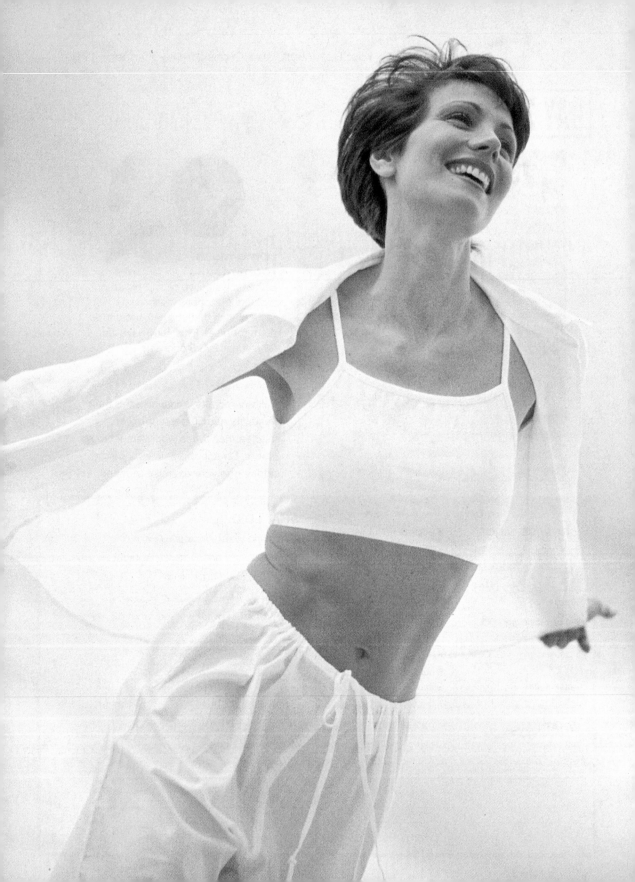

Part 3

Shape-Up Success— Guaranteed

Chapter 9

Look 5 Pounds Thinner Instantly

From office wear to evening wear, look and feel great with these slimming styles.

You can drop 5 pounds in 5 minutes—with the right clothes, that is.

When you know what to wear and how to wear it, you can look slimmer instantly—whether you've just started your shape-up program or you've been exercising diligently and you still have a few inches to lose. You'll not only look great, you'll feel great, too. And that makes it even easier for you to banish your belly, butt, and thighs.

We asked fashion experts what they would wear if they were trying to look slim. They shared their fashion secrets that will help you cover up your belly, elongate your thighs, and smooth out your bottom. From everyday casual wear to elegant styles for a night on the town, follow these tricks of the trade, and you're sure to be turning heads.

Everyday Clothes That Flatter

Whether out with friends or in the office, good casual wear should be flattering—and comfortable.

You want: Tummy coverage, especially if you're wearing pants or a skirt that contrasts with your top or has a high waistband.

Look for: An A-line top to layer over a tapered skirt or straight-leg pants. Try a trapeze top, made in stretchy or gently flowing fabric and worn long, so if you stand with your arms at your sides, it falls somewhere between your fingertips and your knees.

You want: Pants that minimize the appearance of your tummy, hips, and thighs.

Look for: Flat-front pants that minimize bulges with as little fabric as possible. If you like to wear pants with pleats, look for either a quality lining or extended pocket bags. These will prevent your tummy from pulling open the pleats.

You want: A skirt that accommodates a protruding derriere or heavy thighs when worn with a straight, tailored jacket.

Look for: A tapered skirt, which is cut generously through the hips, with a tailored waistband, fitted front, flat front pleats, tapered hem, and back slit. Look for a skirt that's tapered slightly from hip to hemline. The converging lines will narrow and elongate your figure. You'll look slimmer without compromising comfort.

You want: A skirt that diverts attention from your hips, thighs, and tummy.

Look for: A sarong skirt—a skirt with an additional panel of fabric that wraps around the front of your body and ties at one side. The

Shape Up with Shapewear

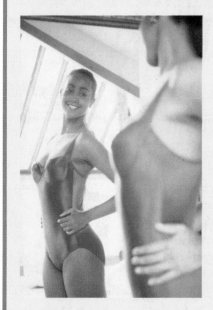

If you add only one item to your wardrobe this year, make it a piece of shapewear: combination bras and panties and other one-piece undergarments that hold you in—comfortably. Nothing takes off as many pounds and firms up so many areas in just seconds. These slimming products include hip slips, full-body slips, long- or high-leg briefs, and even panty hose.

Unlike girdles of old, the new shapewear is comfortable. Choose light, medium, or firm control. Even if you need firm control, the fabric is soft and pliable, and hems often stay in place without thick, stiff elastic that impedes circulation. Look for allover control, with panels at the thighs and tummy to smooth and flatten these areas.

second front fools the eye into thinking the extra fullness comes from your skirt, not your tummy.

FAT BLASTER

Be bold. An interesting top or jacket can divert attention away from the tummy, butt, and thighs. Wear tops embellished with bright colors, beads, or textured fabric.

Office Wear That Suits Your Figure

Casual Fridays aside, tailored pants, skirts, and jackets are still the unofficial uniform for many working women. Experts agree that in order for you to look effective and professional, your office wear must fit perfectly. If your only trouble

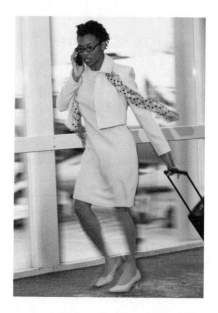

spot is your tummy, you'll have an easier time. But if your body is pear- or hourglass-shaped, it's difficult to find ready-to-wear suits that fit well.

A woman who has a prominent derriere and

Real Women SHOW YOU HOW

The Dress for Success

In her late twenties, Dinah Burnette put on 100 pounds in 2 years. It wasn't until she saw photographs of her 1996 nursing school graduation that she realized just how much weight she'd gained. So she began fixing healthy meals, drinking a gallon of water a day, and exercising regularly. The key to her motivation: A little black dress she'd worn to a wedding in 1989. "I would try it on every 4 weeks to see how close the buttons were getting." One year later and 100 pounds lighter, she could fit into it with room to spare.

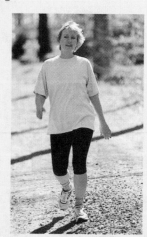

Restyle Your Eating Style

Here are some common yet self-defeating food mindsets, along with refocusing strategies from experts in weight control. Use their suggestions to make over your food attitude.

Old attitude: "All I have to do is tell myself not to eat so much."

New attitude: "I'm going to make some changes in my food milieu: what I buy, where I store food, how I prepare meals, where I eat, what I do while I'm eating, and how I order at restaurants."

Cultivating a new food attitude means making meaningful food decisions, not relying on willpower to avoid temptation, says Kelly Brownell, Ph.D., director of the Yale University Center for Eating and Weight Disorders, who developed the LEARN (Lifestyles, Exercise, Attitudes, Relationships, and Nutrition) Program for Weight Control at the LEARN Education Center in Dallas. In his program, Dr. Brownell tells people to plan their meals, shop from a list, and go to the store on a full stomach—time-honored strategies that work.

"If your refrigerator resembles a salad bar because you shopped wisely, you'll suffer only minor damage if your resolve weakens," Dr. Brownell points out.

Other suggestions from Dr. Brownell include:

▶ Do nothing else while you eat.
▶ Eat on schedule.
▶ Eat in one place.
▶ Do not clean your plate.

Old attitude: "The holidays are coming (or the office bash, a cousin's wedding, or other food fest), so there's no point in even trying to watch what I eat right now."

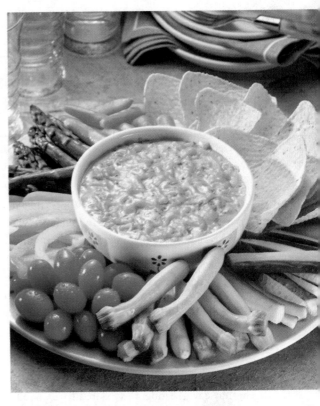

New attitude: "I'm going to develop coping strategies for tempting situations."

"Don't make excuses, take control!" urges Laurie L. Friedman, Ph.D., deputy director of the Johns Hopkins Weight Management Center in Baltimore. Going to a holiday get-together? Offer to bring a salad, a lower-calorie appetizer or dessert, or even an exotic fruit plate. That way, you won't binge on cheesecake because you had no choice, she says. If you choose to eat some cheesecake, eat a small portion and enjoy it. But never let yourself be at the mercy of food or the situation.

"At a buffet, I suggest that people walk through and really look at everything before choosing. Just select a few things that are most appealing," Dr. Friedman says.

Old attitude: "Starting today, I will never eat chocolate (or french fries, or cheeseburgers, or Bavarian cream pastries) again."

New attitude: "I can still eat whatever I want—occasionally. I just need to set limits for myself and stick to them."

Every indulgence doesn't have to turn into a binge, says Dr. Friedman. "Some women may have foods that they like a lot or that trigger a binge for them," she notes. "While they're trying to lose weight, I ask them to temporarily avoid certain foods that might undermine their efforts. But vowing to avoid french fries forever is an empty promise.

"The long-term goal is moderation," Dr. Friedman adds, noting that for many people, high-fat foods lose some of their appeal once they get used to eating healthier choices.

Old attitude: "Well, of course I ate a carton of ice cream at the end of a perfectly healthy day of eating. I'm a slob, I have no self-control, and I deserve to look this way."

New attitude: "No one is perfect. I'm going to think about why this happened, take steps to prevent it the next time, and give myself a break."

Don't fall into what Dr. Brownell calls lightbulb thinking, telling yourself that you are either perfect, eating healthy foods in reasonable portions, or horrible, slipping up and eating a big piece of cake—in essence turning the light out on your whole effort.

Instead, put your slipup in perspective: Over the course of a month, one 2,000-calorie mistake will not make much difference.

The real danger lies in heaping guilt and despair on yourself because you're not perfect, says Dr. Brownell in his LEARN program. If that happens, most likely you'll react by eating even more.

Old attitude: "I'm just going to follow the high-protein, low-carbohydrate diet that worked for my boss. I know it's a fad, but she lost weight really fast."

New attitude: "I need to identify my own food attitudes and plan strategies that work best for me."

Forget the high-protein diet—or any fad diet. Experts emphasize that any diet that eliminates certain food groups and depends heavily on others is unwise from a nutritional standpoint. It also does nothing to help you foster realistic eating patterns.

To do that, says Dr. Brownell, "evaluate your strengths and weaknesses and choose foods and cooking techniques that help you the most." Begin by keeping a food diary of everything you eat for a week. Tally the calories and divide by 7 days. Be sure to take note of the time, what you are doing while you eat, and what you are feeling.

Write it down.
A food diary will help you identify
"automatic" eating habits,
such as munching mindlessly, even when you're **not hungry** and not really appreciating the food.

A food diary will help you identify "automatic" eating habits, such as munching mindlessly, even when you're not hungry and not really appreciating the food. By paying attention to your eating, you'll also be able to spot patterns that may be thwarting your efforts to lose weight, says Raymond C. Baker, Ph.D., a psychologist at the St. Francis Medical Center in Peoria, Illinois. He studied 38 dieters to see who gained and who lost weight from late November through the New Year. The people who monitored their diets most closely lost the most weight. Those who monitored their diets the least actually gained weight, even though they were enrolled in a weight-loss program.

"Be your own scientist," urges Dr. Baker. "See what works for you." He notes that many people who maintain weight loss continue their monitoring over the long haul, for a year or more. That way, they see patterns over time, rather than dwelling on one bad day or one great week.

Old attitude: "I'm under a lot of stress now. I'll eat more sensibly when things calm down."

New attitude: "Things may never calm down. I have to find other ways to cope besides food."

Dr. Baker encourages people enrolled in his weight-control program to stop to analyze the real emotion behind the stress. Are they bored when they eat? Angry? Overwhelmed? Sad?

Ask yourself the same questions. Once you decide what's bothering you, you'll be able to find better alternatives to munching the feeling away, says Dr. Baker. If you're overwhelmed, take time to get organized instead of racing for the doughnut box. If you're sad, think of non-food ways to soothe yourself: You might run a hot, candlelit bath sprinkled with lavender while you listen to music. If you're angry, take a run or a brisk walk.

For handling ongoing or long-term stress, experts recommend learning meditation or deep-breathing techniques.

Old attitude: "I know women who stay slim because they exercise all the time and eat big plates of bulgur, tofu, and other beans and grains. But that's not for me."

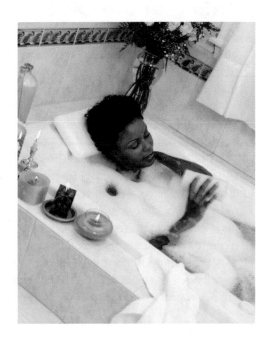

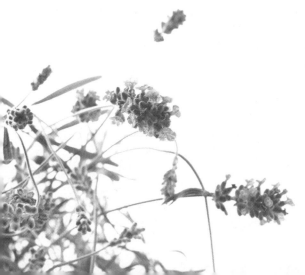

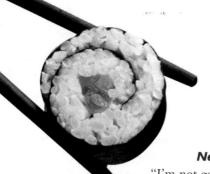

calorie, low-fat food—might change their minds if they try a vegetarian version.

"One suggestion I give almost everybody is to buy one thing you haven't tried before every time you go to the grocery store," Busch says.

Beyond new choices, you may be underestimating the number of healthy foods that you already like, says Anne Dubner, R.D., a registered dietitian and nutritional consultant in Houston.

Every food group contains many, many choices. So if you hate bulgur and cottage cheese, eat whole wheat bread and a low-fat pudding cup instead.

New attitude: "I'm not going to eat foods I hate, but I will try new things. Making healthy lifestyle choices is fun, and doing something good for myself is satisfying."

Visit alternative grocery stores on sampling days and try just a nibble of the week's free offerings, suggests Felicia Busch, R.D., a registered dietitian in St. Paul, Minnesota. People who might cringe at the thought of eating raw fish in the form of sushi—a low-

Old attitude: "I see women who can eat anything they want and still stay skinny as a rail. I'm short, and I gain weight when I just think about food. It's not fair."

Eating at the Office

Almost every workplace has a goody table where people leave cakes, cookies, candy, and pies. For many, sharing food is a big part of work camaraderie. That companionship is so strong that some women fear that their office mates will shun them if they turn down sweets.

To make sure that office eating doesn't sabotage your new body, develop a take-charge approach. What would happen if you proposed to your chocolate-loving buddies that you all embark on a month of healthy eating? "Sometimes other people in the group are struggling, too," says Raymond C. Baker, Ph.D., a psychologist at the St. Francis Medical Center in Peoria, Illinois. Under your plan, you could still share the cooking and eating elements of your friendship without having to sacrifice something important to you—getting in shape. Maybe you could have a potluck soup and salad night, or make healthy box lunches to trade on your break.

Also, give your friends and work pals some credit. If they care about you, they'll want the best for you. Explain your reasons for wanting to make some changes and ask for their help. You may be surprised at their warm response.

Real Women SHOW YOU HOW

A Party Motivated Her to Lose 135 Pounds

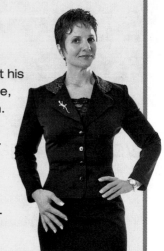

When Sonia Turner, 44, refused to join her husband at his office Christmas party because of her 285-pound frame, the pain in his eyes made her determined to trim down. Sonia started a scrapbook of photos of people exercising, stories of folks overcoming adversity, and a picture from that same Christmas party showing a slim and smiling couple. By the time the next Christmas rolled around, Sonia's healthier eating and exercise habits had pared off 135 pounds, and she and her husband danced the night away at the annual office party.

New attitude: "I'm going to concentrate on looking and feeling my best and stop dwelling on things I can't change."

"If you're destined to be a round person, you're never going to be a skinny-minny, Twiggy-type person," Dubner says. You can exercise and eat healthy foods, however, to make your figure proportionate and firm. As a bonus, you can also keep your heart healthy and your bones strong.

Don't compare yourself to the slender woman eating the overstuffed corned beef sandwich and fries, warns Dubner. "You don't know how much she exercises. Maybe that's the first meal she's eaten all day, and that's not very healthy."

Old attitude: "I lost 50 pounds. Now I can finally eat anything I want."

New attitude: "My new food attitude is a healthy and productive one. Sure, I can indulge in a special dessert once in a while, but my switch to healthy eating is something I'll stick with for a lifetime."

"If you gained weight in the first place, you're prone to gaining it back again," says Dubner. The "I'm fixed now" syndrome is the biggest reason people regain weight, no matter how thrilled they were to reach their goals.

Stick with your food diary and study it periodically to find your vulnerabilities. If you never really shook loose of that late-night snack, make sure you've stocked your kitchen with popcorn and pretzels. "Sometimes, it's much easier to change the food than it is to change the behavior," Dubner notes.

Chapter 11

Stick-with-It Tips for Getting Lean

Follow these, and you'll never skip a workout again.

Okay, you're convinced: Getting some form of calorie-burning exercise a couple of times a week is the best way you're going to leave unwanted pounds behind. The question is, just *when* is all this exercise going to take place? Experts agree: Finding time—and staying motivated—takes some work.

"After a long day at work, it's easier to plop down in front of the TV than to go out for a run or walk," says Joyce Nash, Ph.D., a clinical psychologist in San Francisco and Menlo Park, California, and author of *The New Maximize Your Body Potential*.

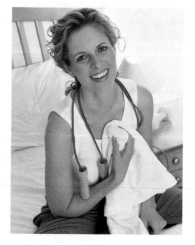

The key to success is to anticipate problems, says Judith Young, Ph.D., executive director of the National Association for Sports and Physical Education in Reston, Virginia. "Identify the things that can prevent you from following through on your plans and make plans for dealing with them," she says.

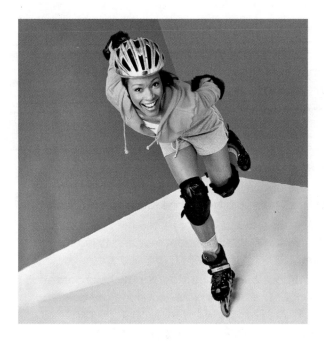

Opt for belly dancing, elliptical training, **inline skating**—or just plain walking, **if that's your pleasure.**

Here's a list from the experts of the top exercise obstacles—with practical tips for countering each.

Problem: You hate to exercise.

Solution: Choose activities that you really, truly enjoy.

Just because your sister-in-law runs, your neighbor goes for marathon bike rides, and your pals at the office go to aerobics classes religiously doesn't mean you have to. Opt for belly dancing, elliptical training, inline skating—or just plain walking, if that's your pleasure, say experts.

Problem: You exercise every day for the first week then get distracted, and by week three, you've abandoned exercise altogether.

Solution: Start out exercising just twice a week. This leaves room for you to have a desire to do more, instead of setting yourself up for failure because you haven't fulfilled greater ambitions.

Problem: Your family needs you. The kids complain when you're not available.

Solution: Include your family in your exercise.

Need some ideas?

► Join a health club that offers babysitting services or kids' activities. You get your exercise while your child gets entertained.

► Do your workout during your child's soccer or softball practice, suggests Dr. Young. Instead of just daydreaming on the bench, walk, jog, or bike.

► Use your small ones as exercise aids, says Dr. Young. Plop your seated infant at your feet and do curl-ups toward her, saying "peek-a-boo" as you sit up. Or sit in a chair, balance your toddler astride your ankles and shins, hold her hands, and bounce her gently up and down, working your quadriceps, she suggests.

Find Exercise Time

Want the definition of the word *busy*? Look at any woman's schedule. So trying to squeeze in exercise may seem next to impossible. But we've come up with six fun and easy ways for you to fit in a workout without stealing any more of your time than you have to.

- Make exercise appointments. Write them down in your daily planner or stick a reminder on your refrigerator door. Fit other appointments around your exercise session, rather than vice versa.
- Do it for 10 minutes. Studies have shown that accumulating 30 minutes of daily exercise in 10-minute chunks has positive calorie-burning and heart-strengthening effects.
- Walk 10 minutes before work, do another 10 at lunchtime, and finish the day with 10 minutes after dinner.
- Exercise with short videos. A number of exercise videos now incorporate a week's worth of short—no longer than 15 minutes—routines on the same tape.
- Walk around the block while dinner's cooking instead of waiting for the meat loaf to bake.
- Make phone calls on a speaker or portable phone while you're on a tread-mill or bike or doing a stretching routine.

Problem: Your family doesn't seem to mind if you exercise, but you still feel guilty when you leave them to work out.

Solution: Tell yourself that you deserve some time to take care of your body.

Consider yourself a positive role model for your children, Dr. Young says. Your routine will demonstrate the benefits of exercise, from having more energy to being in a better mood. Emphasize the concept further still by taking your child along on walks and bike rides.

Problem: You work in an office all day and can't seem to fit in any exercise.

Solution: Be creative and flexible.

Finding time in your day just needs a little inspiration. Try the following:

▶ Work out flexible work hours, recommends Lisa Hoffman, an exercise physiologist and personal trainer in New York City. Arrange for a later starting time so that you can hit the gym before work or for an earlier starting time so you can exercise after work. Or extend your workday so you can take a long lunch break for exercise.

▶ Exercise in your office. Close the door and do crunches or pushups, says Liz Neporent, an exercise physiologist and president of Plus One Health Management in New York City. If you don't have privacy, do exercises in your chair like "writing the alphabet" with your toes, which works your shins and calves. Trace each letter from A to Z on the floor with the big toe of each foot. You can also strengthen your thighs by tightening and releasing your thigh muscles while sitting.

Problem: You have trouble staying motivated when you exercise alone.

Solution: Make exercise time social time.

The more the merrier, even when it comes to working out. Improve your social life and your health with these tips.

▶ When a friend asks you to a movie or dinner, suggest that you go for a hike together instead.

▶ Get an exercise buddy. Working out alone can be a welcome break, but sometimes making a commitment to work out with someone else makes it more likely that you'll actually do it, says Dr. Young. Choose someone who is convenient, such as a neighbor down the block, and who has similar exercise interests and skill levels.

▶ Have an online buddy. If you have computer access to the Internet, send e-mail messages about your workouts to online exercise buddies.

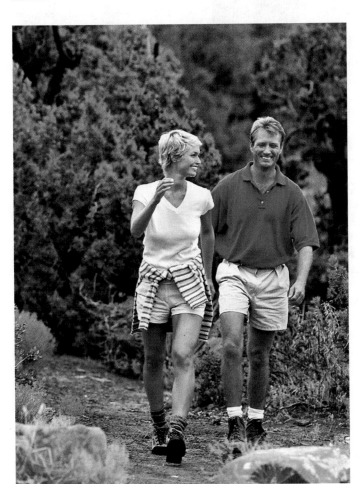

When a friend asks you to a movie or dinner, suggest that you **go for a hike** together instead.

Problem: You can't afford a lot of expensive equipment, gym fees, or fancy workout clothes.

Solution: Keep it simple.

Exercise doesn't have to be expensive. In fact, it's the cheapest form of entertainment out there.

▶ Take up something simple like walking, jogging, or using exercise videos, says Neporent.

▶ Join a gym where you can pay per month or per session. Then go only when you need to—like when it's too cold to exercise outdoors.

▶ Ask for workout clothes instead of other gifts for your birthday, Christmas, Hanukkah, or other special occasions. The same goes for exercise gear like water aerobics aids, aerobic videos, a gel seat for your bicycle, and so forth.

Problem: You'd like to go to the gym, but it's just too much trouble to drive there, especially in bad weather, so you often end up skipping your workout.

Solution: Exercise at home.

Turn your abode into your own "Home Sweet Health Club" with a few simple steps.

▶ A motorized treadmill, stationary bicycle, or exercise video will do just fine for aerobic exercise, says Hoffman. And you can do your workouts to trim your abdominals, hips, thighs, and buttocks at home on a mat.

▶ To create the feel of a health club and help you to keep an eye on your form, add a mirror to your workout space, suggests Neporent.

Real Women SHOW YOU HOW

Fitting in Workouts on the Phone

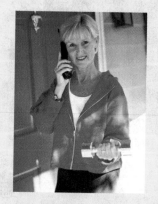

When Jeri Jefferis, now 57, left her job as a phys ed instructor, she worried about regaining the 30 pounds she had lost once before. She was hard-pressed to find time to work out, so she sneaked in some movement whenever she could. While chatting on the phone or being put on hold, Jeri paced the floor or did squats or leg lifts. "If I hadn't started doing that," attests Jeri, "I know I'd have a weight problem today." Every little bit helped, and Jeri has managed to stay trim in spite of her demanding life and career change.

Problem: Your hair and makeup get messed up when you exercise, and you have to go back to work.

Solution: Dealing with perspiration will solve both problems.

Paula Begoun, makeup artist and author of *Don't Go Shopping for Hair Care Products without Me,* says that perspiration makes frizzy hair frizzier and straight hair limp. It also can cause makeup to move and streak. Further, salt from sweat gets trapped under makeup, irritating your skin.

To help your hair, pull it back to get it off your sweaty neck, says Begoun. This will keep you cooler, and your hair will be less likely to get wet, which can destroy just about any hairdo.

As for your face, avoid wearing makeup during exercise, suggests Begoun. The combination of makeup and perspiration may irritate your skin. If you don't want to remove and reapply your makeup for a quick lunchtime workout, use a "stay-put" makeup, which doesn't drip or move. Then, to prevent streaks, gently dab perspiration with a soft cloth as you exercise.

Problem: You mean to work out, but you forget your workout clothes half the time, or you're too rushed to get your exercise gear together before leaving for work.

Solution: Try planning ahead. Pack your workout clothes a day in advance or have extra workout clothes stashed in your desk at work, says Hoffman.

Problem: You start out with enthusiasm, but you just can't seem to stay motivated.

Solution: Remind yourself why you're doing this.

Can't remember why you started? Try these reminders.

▶ Put your reasons down on paper. Write down both the benefits of exercising and getting

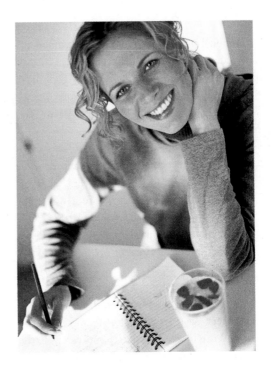

Writing down the
benefits of exercise
and posting them on your
mirror will **help you stay
motivated.**

in shape and the costs of not doing so, suggests Dr. Nash. For example: "Benefit of exercising: I look better in my clothes. Cost of not exercising: I feel fat, tired, and bad about myself." Display your list in a prominent place.

▶ Mentally rehearse doing exercise. What your mind believes, your body achieves, says Dr. Nash. When you wake up in the morning, spend a few moments in bed mentally picturing yourself exercising. Surround yourself with inspirational posters and pictures of women involved in various forms of exercise.

▶ Note your progress. You'll feel more motivated if you check your progress against your initial goals every 2 months or so, says Neporent.

▶ Train for an ambitious goal. Once you're in the swing of regular exercise, pump up your motivation by aiming for an event, suggests Hoffman. For example, if you're a walker or runner, sign up for a local 5-K or 10-K race.

Problem: Some days exercise feels easy, but sometimes, it's a real effort for you to get through.

Solution: Expect tough days and deal with them. It happens to even the most avid of exercisers, says Hoffman. One day you run around the block effortlessly and carefree, the next you count every minute and feel like you're carrying a bag of cement on your back. Expect the mentally tough days and just do your best to push yourself through them, knowing that tomorrow is another day. If you are slowed by a physical (rather than a mental) soreness, however, take it easy, she adds.

Problem: You've been exercising for months, but you're getting bored, and you can't get excited about activities you used to enjoy.

Solution: These are signs that your exercise regimen is getting stale, say experts.

To renew your interest in exercise:

▶ Change the scenery. If you usually work out indoors, logging miles on a treadmill or stationary bike, move your workout outside for a new environment, suggests Dr. Young.

▶ Take up an entirely new activity. If you've always stuck to solitary pursuits, sign up for a team sport, such as volleyball, or a partner game, such as tennis. Or sign up for a class to train for running a marathon.

▶ Try an occasional "take it to the max" workout: If you always do 25 crunches, aim for as many as you can short of muscle cramps, says Dr. Young. If you jog, go to a local track and run a mile as fast as you can, timing yourself with a stopwatch.

▶ Try new exercise toys. Heart-rate monitors, exercise tubes and rubber bands, exerballs, and aquatic exercise gear can make workouts more fun and challenging. Find out which new training gadgets are available for your favorite activity, or try something altogether new with them.

FAT BLASTER

Give yourself a gold star. Using a calendar that displays a month at a time, apply an adhesive gold star for every day that you exercise. Or use a variety of stickers to designate different activities, like happy faces for bike rides and stars for speed-walking.

Credits

Cover photographs

Hilmar

Interior photographs

Artville: page 179

Patricia Brabant-Cole Group/PhotoDisc: page 190

Thomas Brummett/PhotoDisc: page 148

Nancy R. Cohen/PhotoDisc: page 149

Courtesy of Concept II: page 105

Tim De Frisco/Rodale Images: pages 87, 91

EyeWire Collection: pages 62, 65, 66, 69, 165, 173, 176, 184 (woman)

Catherine Gatens/Liaison Agency: page 191

Robert Gerheart/Rodale Images: page 16

John Hamel/Rodale Images: pages 97, 109, 119, 122, 130, 172

Hilmar: pages v (woman eating watermelon and woman eating cereal), x, xi, 2, 9, 12, 15, 29, 34, 36 (Linda Snyder), 54, 56 (Brooke Myers), 59, 64, 89, 111, 125, 136, 138, 139, 143, 144, 145, 146, 150, 154, 155, 156, 157, 158, 159, 160, 161, 162, 163, 166, 168, 170, 174, 178, 182, 186, 192, 193, 195, 196 (Jeri Jefferis), 197

Courtesy of ICON Health and Fitness: page 75

Michael Keller/The Stock Market: page 180

Ed Landrock/Rodale Images: pages 94, 101, 107, 116

Mitch Mandel/Rodale Images: pages 22, 35, 36 (recipe), 38, 39, 40, 43, 44, 47, 49, 50 (recipe), 52, 53, 134, 140, 142, 152, 164, 187

Ryan McVay/PhotoDisc: pages iv (woman jumping rope), v (present), 99, 196 (present)

Courtesy of Precor: page 81

Rodale Images: pages xii, 3, 4, 5, 6 (tea), 10, 13, 14, 21, 24, 26, 27, 28, 31, 32, 37, 42, 46, 51, 55, 56 (pear), 57, 58, 60, 61 (blueberries), 113, 151, 153, 169, 171, 177, 183, 189 (woman)

John Sterling Ruth: page 167

Margaret Skrovanek/Rodale Images: pages 61 (woman), 84

Sally Ann Ullman/Rodale Images: page 128

Tad Ware and Co./Rodale Images: pages 41, 48

Karl Weatherly/PhotoDisc: page 72

Jimmy Williams: page 184 (Dinah Burnette)

Kurt Wilson/Rodale Images: pages iv (nuts), 8, 19, 25, 30, 33, 45, 78, 175, 188, 189 (lavender)

Will Yurman/Liaison Agency: page 50 (Teresa Tomeo)

Interior illustrations

Karen Kuchar: pages 135, 141

Conversion Chart

These equivalents have been slightly rounded to make measuring easier.

Volume Measurements

U.S.	Imperial	Metric
¼ tsp	–	1 ml
½ tsp	–	2 ml
1 tsp	–	5 ml
1 Tbsp	–	15 ml
2 Tbsp (1 oz)	1 fl oz	30 ml
¼ cup (2 oz)	2 fl oz	60 ml
⅓ cup (3 oz)	3 fl oz	80 ml
½ cup (4 oz)	4 fl oz	120 ml
⅔ cup (5 oz)	5 fl oz	160 ml
¾ cup (6 oz)	6 fl oz	180 ml
1 cup (8 oz)	8 fl oz	240 ml

Weight Measurements

U.S.	Metric
1 oz	30 g
2 oz	60 g
4 oz (¼ lb)	115 g
5 oz (⅓ lb)	145 g
6 oz	170 g
7 oz	200 g
8 oz (½ lb)	230 g
10 oz	285 g
12 oz (¾ lb)	340 g
14 oz	400 g
16 oz (1 lb)	455 g
2.2 lb	1 kg

Length Measurements

U.S.	Metric
¼"	0.6 cm
½"	1.25 cm
1"	2.5 cm
2"	5 cm
4"	11 cm
6"	15 cm
8"	20 cm
10"	25 cm
12" (1')	30 cm

Pan Sizes

U.S.	Metric
8" cake pan	20 × 4 cm sandwich or cake tin
9" cake pan	23 × 3.5 cm sandwich or cake tin
11" × 7" baking pan	28 × 18 cm baking tin
13" × 9" baking pan	32.5 × 23 cm baking tin
15" × 10" baking pan	38 × 25.5 cm baking tin (Swiss roll tin)
1½ qt baking dish	1.5 liter baking dish
2 qt baking dish	2 liter baking dish
2 qt rectangular baking dish	30 × 19 cm baking dish
9" pie plate	22 × 4 or 23 × 4 cm pie plate
7" or 8" springform pan	18 or 20 cm springform or loose-bottom cake tin
9" × 5" loaf pan	23 × 13 cm or 2 lb narrow loaf tin or pâté tin

Temperatures

Fahrenheit	Centigrade	Gas
140°	60°	–
160°	70°	–
180°	80°	–
225°	105°	¼
250°	120°	½
275°	135°	1
300°	150°	2
325°	160°	3
350°	180°	4
375°	190°	5
400°	200°	6
425°	220°	7
450°	230°	8
475°	245°	9
500°	260°	–